STRESS MANAGEMENT THROUGH MIND ENGINEERING

STRESS MANAGEMENT THROUGH MIND ENGINEERING

R. P. BANERJEE

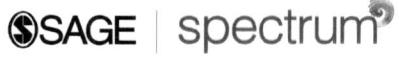

Los Angeles | London | New Delhi
Singapore | Washington DC | Melbourne

First published in 2022 by

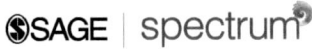

SAGE Publications India Pvt Ltd
B1/I-1 Mohan Cooperative Industrial Area
Mathura Road, New Delhi 110 044, India
www.sagepub.in

Typeset in 9.5/11.5 pt Century Schoolbook.

Library of Congress Control Number: 2021950328

ISBN: 978-93-5479-314-1 (PB)

This book is dedicated

to

the spirit of goodness and

the cause of well-being

सर्वेभवन्तुसुखिनः

सर्वेसन्तुनिरामयाः।

CONTENTS

PREFACE

Complexity and problems are usual associates of life. These have become more important in the context of post-modern world. Left to oneself in an individual context, a person experiences the problems of loneliness. When in the mid of many, the problems arising out of the non-conformity asymmetricism of thoughts create dissatisfaction in the lives of people who participate in the mix of many. It is important that a human being experiences things as designed and desired. The problem that remains is departures from those positions of designs and desires. Whether it is a case of non-conformity, asymmetry in thoughts or departures from the designs/desires, the effect contributes to the incidence of dissatisfaction or depression. This tends to create stressful situations in the minds of individuals.

A work on the subject of stressless mind requires the personal involvement of an individual in cultivating aspects of the mind that would create an autonomous condition. The idea first came from the participants of a workshop conducted by the author on the subject. The entire module has been experienced by this author over a long period. Thus, the concept of being experiential has a proven strength of effectiveness. Besides the experiential part of it, the available approaches of managing stress have been given with a view to offer a comprehensive view of the topic as also the various aspects of mind to create a situation where the mind can effectively develop an autonomous position to withstand all impulses and impacts from situations prevailing around.

Thoughts and works can turn neutral to the impacts and impulses from around when the mind attains the power to overcome the factors causing stress in the person. Stresslessness is a condition of mind that remains amid the world yet stands indifferent to the factors of stress. This mind is autonomous in reality and helps other minds to have a similar identity.

Usually, stress takes different shapes and shades at different stages of life. Factors such as lineage, context, situation, character, patterns of behaviour, nature of associations, nature of work, stream of interactions with people, prevailing or expected uncertainties, socio-economic conditions, cultural convictions, nature of transactions with others, influence of domestic/global conditions, consequential evidence of the actions, assumed disasters, loss of faith in oneself, lack of faith in holistic truth, spell of greed, repetitive desires, propensity to anger, depressions of mind, sense of deprivation, lack of love for others, selfishness, high ego, inappropriate expectations, negatively oriented mind and other similar conditions and contexts create and perpetuate stress in human beings. Whatever be the cause or the supportive factors for stress may be, by its very nature, stress is always a killer force within individuality.

A stressful person is prone to the threats of the erosion of the psycho-physical energy of a person. Stress is a silent killer of the intrinsic potentials of a person. A stressless person is untouched by the stressing factors and trauma.

Stress needs prevention to arrest it from capturing the person's psychic space. If it has cropped in a person, its remedy becomes extremely urgent, else it will take the shape of an invisible demon having the power to destroy positive energy inbuilt in the individual.

In this context, managing stress becomes very important, particularly when the stream of global events brings in and almost continuously projecting uncertainties around the shape of the future.

This work attempts to give clarity to the nature of stress. It has clearly explained stress from different aspects and examined its impact on the mind and health of people. The most important aspect of this work is the spiritual orientation of the person. The spiritual dimension has been adequately covered through depictions and categorical analyses of how to prevent stress. The objective is to create stressless mind—a mind that can easily stand out as independent and unaffected by situations, interactions, transactions, consequential impacts or events. Anyone following the methods and steps suggested in this book will surely experience immense strength of making a stressless mind.

ACKNOWLEDGEMENTS

The concept of a stress-free mind is actually universal. Reasons behind getting an impact of stress are so widely varied that they depend on factors connected with personal attributes such as adaptability, patience, tolerance and being in the mid of the world with a sense of equality across the perspective and the positions of the persons in the world. The internal environment as also the external makes a direct contribution towards disruption of the mental poise of a person in any situation whatsoever. However, the fundamental truth and the basic ways to get rid of the stressful situation were uttered by the Vedic sages for the first time in human civilization. The integrity of mind that adheres to the fundamental principles of truth is the best and the most durable option to create a mental autonomy, wherein the person constantly evolves ways and means to face and defeat the challenges of situations which have the power to disrupt the mental autonomy. The Vedic sages of India, in general, have collectively contributed to the concept of integrated mind and, therefore, the first homage and acknowledgement goes to the sources of truth as mentioned and put across by the Vedic sages.

The work required constant support and technical guidance on developing and fine-tuning the contents including the figures, structures, layout and other technological support for making it a finished work for the benefit of getting ready in the form of a book so that the idea gets leverage to have it tested and experienced by deserving and eager persons. From this perspective, I convey profuse thanks to Professor Sudipta Mitra and Mr Lintu Majumder, both colleagues in the academic activities. I also extend my thanks to my wife Smt. Sipra Banerjee, my son Dr Debajyoti Banerjee and my daughter-in-law Dr Dimple Banerjee.

I extend sincere thanks to the members of the editorial and production teams of SAGE and special thanks to Mr Soumyajit Dutta Chowdhury of SAGE, Kolkata, who made the first suggestion and proposal for this publication.

INTRODUCTION

Where does the mind reside? What are its functions? What shall we do with the mind? Can we think of changing the domain of mind? Does the mind create bondage or does it help in liberating the dimensions of a human being? Shall we consider the mind as one of the most important centres of the human system? These are some questions that one might entertain. The questions become more prominent when we consider all these from the point of view of management.

The mind plays a dominant role in the human system. It can make or break a person. It might help a person grow in the way she or he desires and deserves. It may remain fully involved or may work detached. Mind's domain may be the world around or may be the multitude of possibilities most of which could be beyond the natural rational spirit of existence. The mind may remain fixed at a particular point or may go beyond the purview of the rational and natural expectations. It might be the world itself or the sub-domains of the other world. The mind may be engrossed in the rocks of reality or may deluge in the fantasies. It might act and behave empirically or might sink into the realms of spirituality.

The mind has the power to indulge in any kind of thing. It can make a person dwarf or liberate her or him to a great height. Given a chance, it can do a miracle in the areas of action, thought or accomplishment. It does not and cannot work on its own; it has to depend on the guides and drives of the core 'self'. On its own, the mind does not act for a particular function; it has to receive the instructions of the core 'self' or sometimes the thing called 'conscience'.

True to the spirit of its identity, the mind works and walks faster than any organic or psychological fnction. It has the power to embrace anyone and everyone. It can trade a path that otherwise no other function or organ can perform. Basically restless, the mind has the potentiality to settle down and in a poise that binds the aspects of mind in its own drawn or inherited domain. Surely, the domain could be in the realm of the individual or the collective. If the individual is bothered by the emotions stored in mind, she or he has the scope of operating from a plateau transcended or elevated from the frame of reference of her or his own.

Human problems in the collective are very much derived from the individual. It is the role and imperative of the individual to step in the junks of mind with other aspects of life and activity. Organizations are bothered with the problems of negative emotions such as:

- Backbiting
- Greed
- Jealousy
- Sloth
- Envy
- Covetousness
- Corrupt habits
- Stresses
- Strains of the work

These are eternal problems to the collective as also the individual.

The amount of emotional energy that is concerned in the entire action of the corporation is indicative of the value at stake in the organization. Psycho-physical energy that is wasted in the process is not normally taken care of. Steady use of mental energy in the entire process is likely to ensure the effectiveness of the same in the domain of the mind. Surely, it is a problem of the individual as well as the collective. When the individual alone is involved, she or he is likely to be engrossed in the realm of stress.

A mind stuck to a particular realm of emotion is likely to get influenced by the effects of the area. It requires a vehicle to elevate to a height where the effects are all profound. The mind itself can offer tools to remedy likely problems and difficulties. Here is the scope for the mind to remove and reduce the effects of any wrong or unfavourable development to a personality. Managing stress is possible through a continuous process of changing the poise of the mind. This is a process of making the mind cool and calm. The process involves progressive change or transformations of the mind. Ideally, other conditions remaining constant, it would make a significant change in the orientations of the human mind. Thus, we can call it mind engineering. Mind engineering is an art as well as a science. A process of mind engineering can incorporate a lot of changes in the entire realm of the intrinsic emotional environment of an individual.

Given a particular context in the organization, stress can be either prevented or managed through mind engineering. A person does not have the scope to enforce command over the situation or the factors leading to stress, but she or he has the total authority to mould herself or himself. Mind engineering offers an internal tool to exercise control. In the ultimate analysis, it is likely to change the potentials and power of resistance of the individual. Mind engineering cannot change the external situation but can incorporate a perpetual change in the entire scenario. This can also affect the process of developing the internal autonomy of the person doing this.

The question that arises is: How to accomplish this? Mind engineering being a tool specific to an individual can do a lot for the enhancement of the group objective towards eliminating the effects of stress that is there or is likely to be in a future period.

This being the situation, a clear gap exists in the field of managing and preventing stress, which this work has attempted to fulfil. The work offers a process to actually do the mind engineering and also spell out the effects and likely effects of the same.

The work also makes one acquainted with the existing models and approaches of stress management that prevail in both the Eastern and Western worlds.

The application of mind engineering requires sincere devotion of the person to the systems and processes of it as given in the work. Overnight miracles cannot be expected; it works only through consistent initiative and serious effort. The obvious outcome is the creation of a stressless mind.

CHAPTER 1

THE WORLD OF STRESS

A journey in life is a journey of stress. Actions that we initiate can lead to stress when backed by a specific desire of our own. A desireless mind can also lead to stress because of the heartless surroundings. A result-oriented outlook for our business and industry indeed makes the situation rocky. This has been elusively described by one of the greatest poets T. S. Eliot in his great work, *The Waste Land*. Eliot has described life as follows:

> Here is no water but only rock.
> Rock and no water and sandy road.
> The road winding above among the mountains.
> Which are mountains of rock without water.
> If there were water, we should stop and drink.
> Amongst the rock one can't stop, or think.
> Sweat is dry and feet are in the sand.

Eliot's *The Waste Land* catches up with the corporate reality. This describes the truth of the past as well as of the emerging society. We are definitely into rocky land, amid sands all around. Winning and losing the context for business, trade and commerce repeatedly remind us of the rocky, heartless contexts from where we are destined to operate.

At last, amid all multiplicity of the roads, stress is flaunting on us. Win or lose, actions that one initiates bring in the deluge of reactions. So before initiating a cause, one has to be careful about the likely effects. But being in a world that fosters many ugly things with a lot of allurements meant for deviating from the honourable existence, it is not unnatural for a person to take on a lot of stress. Thriving to manage stress becomes a way of life.

In the process of cut-throat competition, the person slips down to foothold of the mountains or either gets lost or scrambles to return somehow, catching up with a fragile straw.

The peak that one wants to conquer disillusions the chaser. Do you want to win? But do you know at what cost? You have to toil head and foot—try. You find your sweets deceiving you and get in absolutely. The rocky heartless situation solidifies and makes you the task master. You are accountable to the world with most of your fortune and destiny, hence in the ascending of the peak. The water of existence sustains you when you toil hard to find it out.

You rise up, to ascend the pick. If you do so, the cost is yours.

You try and try perpetually, to meet your dream and get burnt out. It is what is called jealousy in your workplace which you foment with a view to being a special person, as you are a special entity that you want to be. You create a world of yours wherein the pursuit of attaining the goals and the pursuit of remaining high placing you at your position become the usual pattern of the world. It is the world of yours. The quest for being what you ought to be—the quest for you becoming what you should be—makes a very unusual content to the world. If you want to be what you thought to be, accept the burns, wounds and toils that you deserve to fulfil your needs and wants. Make your survival a reality by following a path that makes you able enough to traverse the way full of chaos and enigma. You seek peace unto all—so that traversing proves easier, smoother and more certain. Your agonies, sufferings and toils do reflect your actions and behaviours. Utter like Thurman (1976) who similarly proclaimed his agonies to get people along for sharing with the griefs and debuts:

> I share with you the agony of your grief.
> The anguish of your heart finds echo in my own.
> I know I cannot enter all you feel.
> Nor bear with you the burden of your pain.
> I can but offer what my love does give.

The strength of caring.
The warmth of one who seeks to understand.
The silent storm-swept barrenness of so great.
This I do in quite ways.
That cn your lonely path.
You may not walk alone.

Whatever be the context, whatever be the realm, whatever be the tree of your fortune, you walk alone creating echo in the hearts of others on the tones and notes of your pain and anguish. The turnaround takes place through a candid offer of love—a kind of love that communicates each with all the warmth that one seeks from others. Obviously, the warmth would be missing when the other side lacks the understanding of the opposite. This happens in a storm-stricken environment when one tries to communicate to others through a set of interactions that would strive to establish poise in the barrenness of life to make life more meaningful and more effective. Love and concern make the person find their all. In the course of the journey that they have undertaken, it becomes a friendly moment when they get the company of others and the rescue to others—a sort of refuse in the heart of others making them feel for all and establishing a world of their choice.

Human beings try to get a position in the society. Through various interactions and means—all dominated by the interacting ego spreading in all directions with their speed—they try to establish themselves. Even the quest for establishing peace and harmony in the system gets lost to the striving of the soul for the fulfilment of ego. The scenario has been rightly expressed by Taittiriya Upanishad. The striving for peace and harmony is revealed here (Easwaran 1987).

May the Lord of day grant us peace.
May the Lord of night grant us peace.
May the Lord of sight grant us peace.
May the Lord of might grant us peace.
May the Lord of speech grant us peace.
May the Lord of space grant us peace.

It is the quest to all-pervading peace, which is felt in its unique kind of situation and interactions.

Peace at work is considered one of the most important parameters of love in life and waving games all life, be it corporate situation
or another situation which is the ultimate objective of all.

It is all-pervading, which requires understanding of all oppo-
sites taking possession in the society in accordance with that.

The trial and turbulence of life lead us to the incidence of the
cause of conflict. Distractions and chaos form the path of each. In
the past, our actions to the initiatives for achievement in life offered
the quality of action undertaken, as an alternative to the system. We
are responsible partly for the maintenance of cause. The longing for
personal achievements forces us to the continuous stream of chaos.
But at the end of the day, shall we ask about it and question the
vertical ego that makes us different from others and question our
actions from the egoless point of view? We may pray to the Lord that
we follow truth and law, voicing the same with Easwaran (1987).

I bow down to Brahman, source of all power.

I will speak the truth and follow the life.

Guard me and my teacher against all harm.

Guard me and my teacher against all harm.

The amount of submission which this leads to is hard to face
and accept by the modern man. When the individual realizes the
Supreme, they understand the subtle presence of how to fulfil
the known being, how to overcome their limit and how to transcend
their own possession? And does how the individual transcends his
ego self? It is the divine, the all-pervading, that makes him great,
honourable and that transcends from the inherent pettiness, chaos
and conflicts of life.

The dilemma and dichotomy of reality in the world are the
causes of all accounts of stress. The answer lies in our taking refuge
in the Brahman. It is due to our ignorance and conservation of
sticking to the realm of ego, the roots of all sorts of miseries for the
world of the human being in particular. Again, the escape is taking
refuge in the Supreme.

Outward orientation, too much of desires and expectations, also
craving for possessions of things, may make a person vulnerable
to stress. It is like making the body conducive to the quick attacks

of the virus or bacteria. Millions of microbes, virus and bacteria are continuously chasing everybody. They take that body as their ground for action and growth where the soil is ready through dilution of the power to configuration. Divine qualities give us integrity, making us unaffected by Stress.

The process thus starts from the conditions of understanding one's hard-pressed context and thereafter aligning one with the expectations to reach the heights of attainment and establishing peace and harmony, alleviating the conditions of burnouts.

STRESS: WHAT IS IT?

Derived from Latin, the word 'stress' was considered to mean things such as hardship, strains, adversities and affliction, according to the early 20th-century editions of Oxford English Dictionary. The meaning of the term 'stress' has undergone rapid changes with the change in the conditions of life and circumstances. During the later stage of the century, stress has been progressively used to mean force, pressure, strain or strong effects. Stress is nowadays considered as a pressure on the personal system and environment of an individual. It is also the demand on the energy system of a person to get certain things done by the person for the entity or the system demanding the aforementioned things.

MEDICAL DEFINITION OF STRESS

In medical terminology, 'stress' has been used to mean things that are on demand for a person, physiologically, psychologically and socially. Medical Dictionary (as quoted in Southerland, 1993) defines stress as:

1. The reactions of the animal body to forces of a deleterious nature, infections and various abnormal states that tend to disturb its normal psychological equilibrium
2. The resisting force set-up in a body as a result of an externally applied force
3. In psychology, a physical or psychological stimulus which, when impinging upon an individual, produces strain or disequilibrium.

In other words, the medical representation of stress has been something that considers the stimuli or responses in a body system involving 'the physical, psychological and social dynamics of the forces applied on it and the necessary build-ups to resist or stop the occurrence of those stimuli'.

STIMULUS–RESPONSE-BASED DEFINITION OF STRESS

The model offered by Cox (1978) discusses stress from the point of view of stimulus–response. According to this model, stress is regarded as an imbalance between the perceived demands made on an individual and the perceived coping ability of the individual. According to this model, if a person does not realize that they cannot cope, they will not be stressed. On the other hand, if they are capable of coping but think that they cannot cope, they will be stressed.

GENERAL ADAPTATION SYNDROME MODEL

The general adaptation syndrome (GAS) model of Selye (1956) has offered another view of stress which contains somewhat medical connotation and takes into account the responses and reactions produced by the somatic system to prevent and stop stress. This approach considers occurrence of non-specific stress that is slowly or abruptly into the individual's personal environment. Selye postulated that in the process of getting stressed, a general level of adaptation takes place. This phenomenon has been identified by Selye as GAS and is understood to have three stages of stressing as mentioned hereunder.

1. **The alarm reaction:** Initially, the level of resistance is poor; however, later on, the individual's defence mechanism becomes active through the process of countershock. This is known as an alarm reaction.

2. **Resistance:** This is the stage of maximum and at times successful return to the equilibrium condition for the individual in a given environment to work with. If, however, the stressor continues to work, the individual might reach a stage or a situation of exhaustion and become a real prey to the system or approaches of stress.

3. **Exhaustion:** When the adaptive mechanism collapses, exhaustion takes place and reaches the maximum height. This is more so when the stressor is continuously recurrent and does not stop.

DEFINING STRESS FROM HOLISTIC VIEWPOINT

So far, we have discussed some of the important models on stress. These include the views of medical scientists, behavioural scientists and management experts. Although the concepts overviewed contain views from diverse angles, 'stress', as the term connotes, means certain things that are intrinsic and certain other things that are extrinsic to human personality.

According to Wolf and Goodwell, stress is a state of the human organism. Wolf and Goodwell suggest that it is an inevitable imperative in the human system; they opine that individuals are continuously in a state of stress. Inherent dynamism in a human system makes a person prone to stress.

According to Lazarus (1971), stress refers to the demands that tax the psychological system and the responses to that. The response or reaction to stress is registered at the cognitive stage and is a function of the individual's response through appraisals of the contents and forms of taxing into the system. So any change in either the external or the internal factors will change the context and content of the thing, thereby changing the meaning and contents of stress.

Certain factors are found common in almost all views on stress. These factors could be summarized as follows:

1. External pressure on an individual causing him ultimate harm and creating problems for him
2. Any kind of harm to the individual making an enduring mark on him
3. An individual's taking stock of the situation and reactive responses to the stimuli.

STRESS: THE HOLISTIC VIEW

Stress has become associated with the modern or postmodern era of living and management. Accept it or not, it exists in the personal life of every individual, society and organization. Today's techno-commercial age, while offering several tools and techniques, has proved ineffective in at least one area—the domain of personal life or the person–system interface where a person becomes an instrument of the system. This is contrary to man's nature, leads to unhealthy situations and is worthy of humane conditionalities. These unnatural and unhealthy things destroy the positive inner substances or elan vital. Stress is a condition of the negative disposition of a human being. The interplay of the vital trio through demands, constraints and supports could be considered as the vital trio in human life and has to be well orchestrated to lead to a balance in life. Whatever be the phase in life, within the limits of one's own activity and scope, one has to establish a balance in the chain of the triangular pull of the vital trio. While demand in life may start in a humble shape, it may culminate into an unrestrained spring that goes on placing one demand after another. One demand of lower order or smaller dimension could be replaced by another with a higher-order or broader dimension. The series of an unending spring of demands thus fails to realize the existence of a halting point—a point that needs reckoning, rethinking and reworking on. There could be cases where the individual, in their surface existence, fails to understand the presence of tangible or formed demand but is compelled to fall under the spell of it. This could be the case of hidden or suppressed demand taking a lead over the 'self' to settle a score without taking into cognizance the reality inside or outside the individual. It could be that the felt need within a very deep layer of the mind sleeps for a long period, awaiting an opening through the surface mind and finds an opportunity to come up having been lit by the ingredients presently available there. It is this mechanism that traps a person in the upsurge of demand from within.

Constraints, unlike demand, could be both inner and outer or either of these two. Constraints put a negative barrier on demand. They could be either from the conscience of the individual, urging him to do something or not do at all, or could be external, imposing some restrictions on his functions and performances. Conscience can put a halt, or at least try to do so, in cases where the thought process or action is engineered by the individual. Conscience can also help the individual a lot to come up and face situations, be it pleasant or not. Sometimes the constraints put or engineered by the conscience appear to be the kind of things that disgust the individual initially but later find ultimate support in its role to save the individual from doing or being involved in unethical acts. Thus, the role of conscience is quite distinct and positive; even then, if it appears unpleasant in the initial phase, it may cause stress.

Supports, like constraints, may also originate from within or from outside. Supports coming from within an individual positively contribute to their future actions and those coming from outside an individual also help them to stand. The question is support for what? Is it for any kind of action or for certain things that pass the tests of 'should or ought'? Unless the drive passes through the tests of 'shoulds' and 'oughts', it can lead to certain kinds of degeneration and finally can lead to a stressful situation. For example, an individual goes ahead at a faster rate if they get support from within and without for any kind of thing. Autocracy develops in such a situation, ultimately culminating in degeneration or destruction through a spell of stress.

Therefore, it appears that demands, constraints and supports may be the active and prominent parameters existing around individuals but may be able to lead to a situation that has deviated from the natural track of an individual's existence. Demand, smoothened by constraint and supported by 'shoulds' and 'oughts', can lead to a situation in which the individual may feel free to act and grow precisely without the feeling of any kind of external pressure. This could be one way of looking into things and events. The other way could be to examine the environment in which one is to work. Is it conducive to health or eating into the vital of individuals? Worries and anxieties in life seem to create cumulative pressure on life to make it stressful. A compelling situation may be bad enough to be stressful. When there is a mismatch between an individual's power and his capability to cope with any given situation, one is thrown into the fire of emotions that sprinkles over the inner mental substance to create a condition called stress.

STRESSOR OR STRESSED: THE DOMINANCE FACTOR

Stress is a kind of perceived pressure on individuals in an organizational context. In the personal domain of an individual, stress is generated and stored in our mind to have an impelling impact on the personality to lead to a situation that is worthy of being called a deranged state of mind. Stress is a situation that finds its place in the human mind and is released through action or counteraction through the vehicles of emotions.

Usually, in an organizational context, the following could be the causative factors:

1. Workload
2. Lack of proper recognition
3. Lack of rewards
4. Work environment
5. People at the top or those around
6. Prevailing customs
7. Organizational culture
8. Fulfilment of material needs

One can go on listing numerous causes for stress and yet find the list incomplete. Stress cannot be conclusively identified with the number of factors causing it. Rather, it would be wiser to conclude that stress may be the result of a dissatisfied ego.

This point could be explained well by discussing the diagram shown in Figure 1.1.

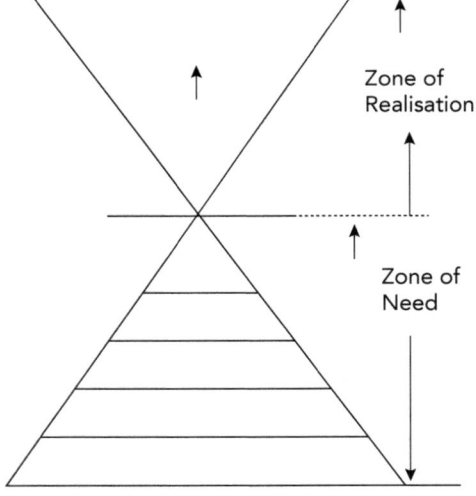

Figure 1.1 Beyond Maslow's Pyramid of Needs

Stress might occur through the denial of any of the needs as shown in the zone of need. A person gets stressed if they do not get fulfilment on the following:

1. Physical needs
2. Safety needs
3. Social needs
4. Esteem needs
5. Self-actualization needs

Human experience has proven the incidence of the next higher-order need on fulfilment of one kind. It is like adding fuel to fire. One quenched need gives birth to another need. When a person reaches the level of self-realization, they remain indifferent to or are unaffected by the current of events. This point of the impact of realization will be discussed later in this book. However, so long as we are unable to reach that height or personality, we remain in the mid of stress. Stress comes through the duality of the world. This duality has got twin dimensions as mentioned below:

1. Copability and capability
2. Need and fulfilment
3. Expectations and provisions
4. Sense of identity and recognition
5. Material wants and material gains
6. Emotional inclinations and physical constraints
7. Philosophy of life and appearance of the world
8. Sense of integrity and impacts of fragmentation
9. Aim and purpose of the individual and that of the whole
10. Philosophy and culture of the individual and that of the organization
11. Truth and reality envisioned by the individual and that of the organization

While the set of above-listed dualities may not be conclusive, they are surely indicative. Stress arises basically out of certain deviations—maybe from one's expectations, concepts, ideas and views of life. A person may feel stressed out if he/she is denied certain things. For example, a person wants a promotion but is denied it. This is a stressful situation for that person.

Before we proceed to elaborate on certain mismatches causing stress, the discussion of some of the prevailing concepts of stress may prove to be useful. Any standard dictionary describes stress as hardship, adversity, affliction, force or pressure exercised by a person for the purpose of compulsion or extortion to oppress. Going by this unique interpretation of the dictionary, one can guess whether the stress is healthy or unhealthy. While healthy stress could lead to a challenging situation, stimulating one's capacity and making one proactive and ready to face situations, unhealthy stress could lead to a decaying situation. The latter is the other side of the challenge and can be termed as stress. When stress fails to generate challenge, it is supposed to lead an individual to a situation called distress.

The variety of stress that is prone to stimulate challenge can be called 'healthy stress', and the other one that leads to distress can be termed as 'unhealthy stress'. For example, hardship and adversity could be identified as the twin factors that can push a person to a combating situation from where the strength and impetus to fight the conditions of hardship and adversity may come. One gets back to the source of hidden treasure within oneself. A person regains self-conviction becoming capable of facing hardships and adversity. This is a case of healthy stress that helps improve a person. There could be situations like being sandwiched by the compelling pressures from different sides. Then one learns a new skill, thus enhancing one's capability to establish a higher-order balance on the scales of copability. A person hardboiled through sandwiching pressures is now capable of facing greater onslaughts in his/her life and can maintain a fair degree of poise during difficult situations. Based on this, it can be said that a person is elevated while passing through a stressful situation. The other example could be a person, towards the end of his career, getting lost by the misbehaviour of a superior or a junior or by denial of legitimate promotion they deserve. Having lost the fruitfulness of the purpose of their working in the said environment, the person may develop a kind of apathy to their job, colleagues and organization. The actions of such individuals tell upon not only the organization but also upon themselves.

The lost sense of purpose and meaning of work may lead to a loss of personal motivation and initiative in general, ultimately ruining the person. Here comes the question of copability. In the case of negative impacts of stress (effects of unhealthy stress), one needs to develop the necessary strength and power to cope with a situation that attempts to destroy the balance both within and without.

WARREN–TOLL'S MODEL OF STRESS

While we try to categorize unhealthy and healthy stress, we find that prevailing views differ widely. This model explains stress (Warren and Toll 1993) as a tightrope that involves three parameters, namely the demand, constraints and supports.

1. A demand made on us
2. Constraints that limit one's capacity to meet the demand and make it seem greater
3. Available supports help us to meet or manage the demand
4. Demands and constraints create pressure
5. The effect on us is stress

Here, the authors, while discussing the process of stress, give more importance to the externals, the constraints and supports imposed upon us or coming from outside. Is it always the external demand made upon us that leads to stress or is it something that is a function of the inner self? We, the individuals, do nurture certain kinds of images and want others to fall in line with that content only. When we discuss impelling demands, we tend to consider them to be more appropriate or more logical. Capability comes next, as an important factor, when we see that in our context, capability or skill come up to match with the situation we have fallen in—putting us in a condition of stress.

   In a relatively recent study, Pestonjee (as quoted in Davies Richard, 1998) has explained organizational stress as a 'situation wherein job-related factors interact in such a way that the worker experiences a disruption in his or her psychological and/or physical conditions so that he is forced to deviate from normal functioning'. This view of Pestonjee takes into account the role of internal factors in creating stress. However, the problem remains as it does not take into account an individual's capability or the power and strength dormant within to face situations that are not favourable to them.

External factors are no doubt countable and important, but more important are the set of internal factors. An individual who is autonomous by faith and conviction can sweep over the external stressing factors more easily than another type of individuals.

Nebeker and Tatum (1993) highlight the scope of capability in work:

'The pattern of findings for satisfaction and stress may indicate that workers become frustrated and demoralized when standards or rewards are high.'

Stress extends a collaborative hand from within; there could be situations when internal stressing factors are present. For example, a person weak in mind, facing pressures from their bosses, adds up to the causative external factors that cause stress, more than the internal ones. The weak mind magnifies stress through a spell of apprehension and defeat. A person, already defeated in mind, finds it important to see the condition where their inherent defeatist attitude is countermanded by an external assurance or support. On the contrary, if pressure mounts on them from outside, their defeatism multiplies to produce a situation of further recoil and the individual caught in such a situation gets lost or they fail to reckon the purpose of their existence. It is not the case of separation or discrimination by time present, time past and time future, or the spatial separation, but the case of the internal potent of a person. Low potent begets lower output and positions a person lower than a person facing stress. It could be a relative situation and could vary from person to person. When we see that an individual working in the present time is most potent for the future, we acclaim them. The individuals also get psychological support in realizing their inner potentiality. But the concept of time becomes important here. The classical views of physical science think the future be separated from the past by an infinitely short interval, the present moment, whereas the relativistic view states that future and past are separated by a finite time interval, the length of which depends on the distance from the observer.

An observer, at a given instant, neither knows nor influences any event at a distant point that takes place between two characteristic times (as quoted in Roger Penrose, 1994). The notion of time vis-à-vis that of potentiality is of great help to us while examining the scope of stress in an individual's life. The twin factors of potentiality and time make the difference between the effects of a common cause through either of them to a person experiencing the cause. Again, I think that an example will help to explain this concept.

Three people are working in the computer room of the railway's city booking counter. Suddenly, a bomb planted by terrorists blasts there. The condition of these three people exposed to the common situation of bomb blast could be different. The person with a weak heart collapses. Another person heaves a deep sigh of relief to manage the heart throbbing, and the third one, with a strong nerve and heart, rushes to the spot and joins work to rescue other people. The quantum of stress generated in all three people as well as the quality of stress is different. In the case of the first two people, it was unhealthy stress, but the action of the third one proves to be a case of healthy stress, converting the stressing factor into challenges and facing the situation.

Another interesting case worth mentioning here is taken from Mathews (1991). This is a real-life case of sexual harassment, a brief presentation of which is as follows.

Jane had joined a company as a secretary to Mike and used to enjoy the work given to her. Mike had given her a project, and Jane finished it in a month of hard toil. But the boss wanted to be on close terms with Jane. She was invited to a day-long bicycle ride; Jane responded favourably but refused to cater to the ugly propositions of her boss. One day Jane found a note with hints of displeasure from the boss on her table. Jane had approached Mike with the note but heard even very direct words of sexual appeals. Jane made sustained efforts to have the matter resolved by the higher authorities but failed to get any positive response. After having failed in all her efforts, Jane found in herself a scattered personality, totally broken due to sexual harassment by her boss.

This case of Jane reminds us of the need for inner strength, poise, power and urges to combat the external stressful factors. An autonomous being, well aware of his or her potentiality, is supposed to be in a better situation to cope with external stress. Stresses, coming from any side—the boss, peers, subordinate groups, political clouts or problems faced in the family—are coped in a better manner if a person learns to manage situations with the strength and conviction of a leader with a motherly heart.

This analysis proves a point that the all-integrative view of stress could be defined as follows: Stress is an outcome of duality that disturbs human equilibrium and creates a negative impact on the human system.

Stress is, obviously, a factor of the dual world and a term with a natural negative connotation on the human system. It is thus against the concept of challenge in the human system. An example from a real-life occurrence can well prove this point.

FACE THE BRUTES

This incident happened to Swami Vivekananda, the founder of the Sri Ramakrishna Order. Vivekananda was chased by a group of monkeys when he was walking towards Durgabari (House of Goddess Durga) across the roads of Benares in India. The first impulse that came in the mind of Swami was to run away which he had resorted to. The monkeys with a feeling of victory had chased him further and more intensely. At this point, a brother monk of Swami Vivekananda who saw the scene from a distance shouted at the Swami telling him to face the brute. In a moment, Vivekananda realized the truth and turned back and faced the monkeys. Immediately after this, the monkeys also turned around and swiftly fled away.

This is an example of converting 'stress' into 'challenge'. As has been indicated, the challenge has a great deal to do with the continuous or discrete flow of vigour and energy into the system. Stress, expressed in simple terms, is the adverse situation in human life where a person ought to face a lot of odds to keep a normal flow of the process of life. This requires a lot of energy, willpower and assertion. An assertive life can have a lot of adverse impositions on it.

This finally converges to a point that man, a psychosomatic being, can win stress to a great extent through conversion of challenging situations and winning that through assertiveness of mind.

MODELS OF STRESS

While defining and presenting stress, we have seen a host of different approaches to stress. The basic impetus may be derived from Aristotle who said of the wise person as those whose choice was not seeking pleasure but freedom from care and pain.

Arthur Schopenhauer, a great philosopher of profound pessimism, had observed the process of life as the process that has been shaped by the desire upon which it is built. Schopenhauer has talked in the same line and spirit of the ancient Indian sage, Manu, on desire. Schopenhauer describes that for every wish that is satisfied, there remain tens of wishes that are denied. 'Desire' is infinite, and fulfilment of desire is only limited. Schopenhauer (Durant 1957) describes this as follows:

> The satisfied passions often lead to unhappiness rather than to happiness. For its demands often conflict so much with the personal Welfare of him who is concerned that they undermine it. Each individual bears within himself a disruptive contradiction; the realised desire develops a new desire and so on, endlessly.

Life is evil because pain is its basic stimulus and reality, and pleasure is merely a negative cessation of pain—Schopenhauer (Durant 1957). This statement can elaborate this basic view expressed in his philosophy in the following words:

> In every individual the measure of pain essential to him was determined once for all by his nature; a measure which could neither remain empty, nor be more than filled.... If a great and pressing care is lifted from our breast ... another immediately replaces it, the whole material of which was already there before, but could not come into consciousness as care because there was no capacity left for it.... But now that there is room for this it comes forward and occupies the throne.

Arthur Schopenhauer's view of life shows the negative and their impacts. The view is further strengthened with a positive inclination by the Existentialist School of Thought. Jean-Paul Sartre defines the current set of interactions as phenomena. According to him, the phenomenon must be understood as a being that reveals itself as it is and as a being that is absolutely indicative of it and refers to nothing but itself. Sartre had said (Grinsley 1967) that 'Every appearance has a transcendant or transphenomenal reference in so far as it refers to other phenomenal aspects which are not given a particular intuition.'

According to Sartre, a being is the basis of nothing and in fact, presupposes it. Nothing can have only a derivative existence. This is because a human being is a freedom seeker. Sartre puts the sequence as follows: 'human freedom precedes the essence of man and helps him to make it possible. Freedom is indistinguishable from the being of human existence. Man does not first of all exist and then become free. He is free. He, himself is freedom.'

The philosophical basis of stress could be well drawn from the concept of a free being. A deviation from the free being changes the equilibrium of the human system in a way that creates situations for stress. A free being, under the pressure of the intrinsic and extrinsic factors, becomes a non-free entity. This is a condition for stress in the system. Stress is generated from a deviation from freedom and could be alleviated through the restoration of integrity and autonomy in the human system.

Various models of stress have been developed by experts based on their views and studies. C. L. Cooper, H. Selye and T. Cox are among experts to develop their models which are worth mentioning and explaining. We shall now discuss some of the models of stress.

Response-based Model of Stress

This model is based on the concepts of John Locke, a 17th-century physician and philosopher. Locke proposed that intellectual functioning, emotion, muscle movement and the behaviour of internal organs are the results of sensory experience produced by the brain. From these early emotions, the field of psychology gradually developed; the links were established between life experiences, emotions and the importance of hormone and chemical actions in the body. Stimulus response is threefold. Responses to all the stimuli have psychological, physiological and behavioural aspects. The model is good at linking various functions but fails to integrate the three functions and

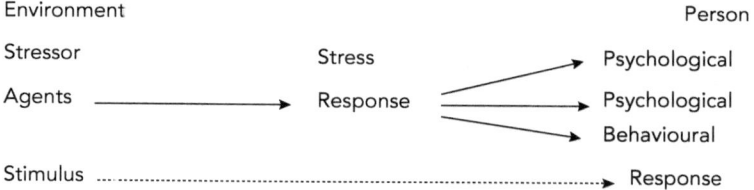

Figure 1.2 Response-based Model of Stress

Source: Southerland and Cooper (1993).

also to show the dominance of one among the three functions. The failure of this model lies further in the basic view upon which the model rests. The fundamental control of all the functioning comes from the domain of the inner self. Independence of the inner self of the influences of the externals makes one stress-free in life, allowing the individual to develop the art and power to resist stress in life.

General Adaptation Syndrome Model

This model is based upon the following key factors:

1. Shock
2. Counterpressure
3. Resistance
4. Collapse

This model recognizes the onset of shock in the entire process of stress. This shock comes from extrinsic factors. Once the shock is felt, the human system develops a counterpressure. The counterpressure grows vigorous and creates a resistance up to the level of beating the system—counterpressure rises to a height for the system to continue, beyond which the scope of counterpressure fades out and finally finds no way out but collapses. Stages 1–4 shown in Figure 1.3 explain this syndrome.

This model is very useful in that it recognizes the process and interactions more vividly. The system relies heavily on the factors of resistance and counterpressure and recognizes the fact that individuals collapse beyond a certain point.

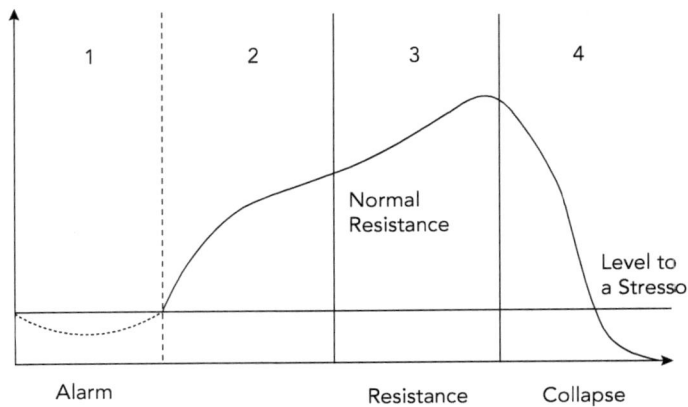

Figure 1.3 General Adaptation Syndrome (GAS)

Source: Selye (1956).

The model fails to understand and identify the real source of counterpressure and resistance. Counterpressure could come from the externals or the intrinsic. It is the inner person or the intrinsic personality which can more reliably manage the shock and take the person to a transcended height to manage stress.

The Health Outcome Model

This model is based on a flow diagram that depicts the interrelationships among cognitive, behavioural and psychological factors as shown in Figure 1.4:

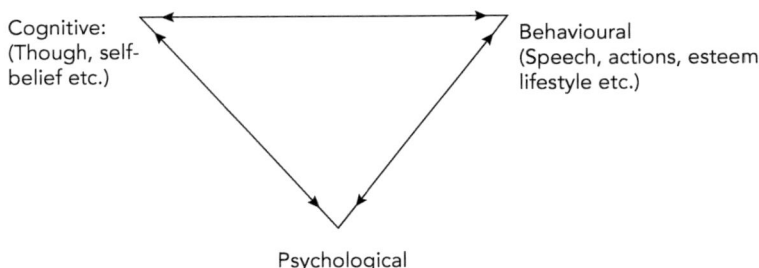

Figure 1.4 The Interactive Nature of Factors in Health Outcome Model

Source: Southerland and Cooper (1993).

Cooper's Model of Stress

Cooper's model of stress discusses different sources of stress at work at five different levels:

1. Intrinsic to the job
2. Role in organizations
3. Career developments
4. Relationships at work
5. Organizational structure and climate

The impact of stress developed at each of the above stages is felt and experienced by the individual. House-work interface is also considered as a major source of stress affecting the individual. The model is essentially a health outcome model with all the actions having the results in terms of the health of the individual. At this point, the World Health Organization's (WHO) definitions of health may be considered. WHO defines 'health' as not only the absence of disease or infirmity but also a state of physical, mental and social well-being (WHO 1984).

By the WHO standards, Cooper's model stands as a health model. All the outcomes are estimated in terms of the physical or mental health standards. The effect on the organization is shown as the total of the understanding of the individuals. Thus, it is seen that organizational impacts are limited to the levels where the formulation of collectives is easier. In this model, high absenteeism and high turnover have been shown in the case of labourers.

The model offers a wider view but lacks the clarity of understanding of the basic process of stress in a human system and the flow of influence showing the relationship of one with the other. The basic drawback of a health outcome model is the lack of confidence in the holistic spirits of the human personality. Stress occurs when the individual deviates from the basic understanding of the holistic potential of individuals. When stress is converted to a challenge, it enters a stream of positive energy to combat and restrict stress.

Transactional or Interactive Model of Stress

This model is again a health outcome model but with some modifications over Cooper's model in terms of individual environment relationships.

Table 1.1 Transactional or Interactive Model of Stress

Environment	Individual	Response	
Potential	Attitudes,	Imbalance = Distress	
Source	Needs, Values,	Pressure or Strain	
of Stress	Past-Experience,		
=Actual	Personality Traits,	Coping	Unable
Demand	etc.	i.e.	to
+	+	Success	cope
Background	Age, Sex, Education		and
and	= Actual Ability		unsuccessful
Situational	Judgement of		
Factors	Threat, i.e., Cognitive	Overcome	
	Appraisal	this problem	Symptoms
	= Perceived Ability		of
	and Perceived Demand Perceived Demand		Stress

Source: Southerland and Cooper (1993).

ANALYSIS OF TRANSACTIONAL OR INTERACTIVE MODEL

This model, as shown in Table 1.1, correlates actual demand to actual ability and perceived demand to the imbalance in the individual's response. The actual ability has been shown as the combination of attitudes, needs, values, past experience, personality traits, etc., and the impacts of age, sex and education. The impact of an individual's potentials has been ignored here. Whereas the actuals are time-variant and environment-variant factors, the potentials do a lot to change the conditions of actuals. Under the impact of the potentials, actuals do change continuously.

There is no doubt that a mismatch between perceived ability and perceived demand creates distress or pressure. To the extent this pressure is sustained and absorbed through coping, stress is less—leaving out the residual distress as stress on the individual.

As has already been mentioned, an analysis of the individual's potential changes the whole arrangement, thus leading to stress. Potentials could be measured at the gross or the perceptible level. Perceptible potential again is founded on the individual's ability to unfold their internal treasures. The underlying belief is that the individual is potentially divine and hence has got the being of his choice, taste and preference through personal efforts and initiatives. As soon as the belief in their being potentially divine is there, the individual grows bigger than their size in terms of internal strengths. They develops a higher power to combat stress. Being in the same stressful situation as in another person, the individual is more fit and assures a happier life than many others.

BIBLIOGRAPHY

Arthur, Koestlesr. 1989. *The Ghost in Machine*. Arkana: Penguin.

Barkow, J. H., I. Cosmides, and J. Tooby, eds. 1992. *The Adopted Mind. Evolutionary Psychology and the Generation of Culture*. New York: Oxford University Press.

Cooper, C. L. 1986. 'Job Distress: Recent Research and the Emerging Role of Clinical Occupational Psychologist'. *Bulletin of the British Psychological Society* 39: 325–31.

Cooper, C. L., and R. Payne, eds. 1990. *Causes, Coping and Consequences of Stress at Work*. New York: John Wiley.

Cox, T. 1978. *Stress*. London: Macmillan.

David, Fontana. 1989. *Managing Stress*. London: The British Psychological Society and Routledge.

Davies, Richard, ed. 1998. *Stress in Social Work*. London: Jessica Kingsley Publishers.

Durant, Will. 1957. *The Story of Philosophy*. New York: Pocket Bocks.

Easwaran, E., Tr. 1987. *The Upanishads*. London: Arkana.

Grinsley, R. 1967. *Existentialist Thought*. Cardiff: University of Wales Press.

James, Earnest. 1977. *Papers on Psycho-Analysis*. London: Maresfield Reprints.

Jeffrey, Alan Gray. 1991. *The Psychology of Fear and Stress*, 2nd edition. Cambridge: Cambridge University Press.

Lazarus, R. S. 1971. 'The Concept of Stress and Disease'. In *Society. Stress and Disease*, edited by L. Levi, Vol. 1. London: Oxford University Press.

Marshall, J., and C. L. Cooper. 1979. *Executive under Pressure: A Psychological Study*. London: Macmillan.

McManus, I. C., and P. Richards. 1992. *Psychology in Medicine*. Amsterdam: Butterworth Heinemann.

Nebeker, Dilbert M., and Charles B. Tatum. 1993. 'The Effect of Computer Monitoring, Standards and Rewards on Work Performance, Job Satisfaction and Stress'. *Journal of Applied Social Psychology* 23: 7.

Newton, T. 1995. *Managing Stress, Emotion and Power at Work*. London: SAGE Publications.

Priest, S., and J. Welch. 1998. *Creating a Stress-free Office, Gower Management Workbooks*. Aldershot: Gower Publishing.

Robert, Feldman S. 1993. *Understanding Psychology*. New York: McGraw Hill.

Roger, Penrose. 1994. *Shadows of the Mind*. Oxford: Oxford University Press.

Selye, H. 1956. *The Stress of Life*. New York: McGraw Hill.

Southerland, V. J., and C. L. Cooper. 1993. *Understanding Stress: A Psychological Perspective for Health Professionals*. London: Chapman and Hall.

Thompson, N., M. Murphy, and S. Standing. 1994. *Dealing with Stress*. London: Macmillan.

Thurman, H. 1976. *Meditations of the Heart*. Richmond: Friends United Press.

Wanda, Nash. 1988. *At Ease with Stress: The Approach of Wholeness*. London: DaVton, Longman and Todd.

Warren, Eve, and Caroline Toll. 1993. *The Stress Workbook*. London: Nicholas Brealey Publishing.

WHO. 1984. *Psychological Factors and Health: Monitoring the Psycho-Social Work Environment and Workers' Health*. Geneva: World Health Organization.

Wolf, H. G., and H. Goodwell. 1968. *Stress and Disease*, 2nd edition. Springfield: C. C. Thomas.

CHAPTER 2

STRESS MANAGEMENT THROUGH INDIAN INSIGHT

INTRODUCTION

Accept it or not, stress exists in life. In the social as well as organizational life, stress is a daily affair. We are under the spell of stress. In a family or an organization, we are the victims of an interplay of demands, constraints and supports. Most of the time, we fail to establish a balance among the trio—the factors of demands, constraints and supports. Occasionally, we remain unaware of the demands we are supposed to fulfil and consequently become an auto-victim of stress. Constrained tightly, sometimes we forget to consider the boundary condition, thereby inviting stress. Lack of legitimate support also leads to stress. Whereas life demands a balance, we are very much prone to the chosen imbalances. The hectic activity from day to day makes our life vibrant but at the same time dynamic and productive. Stress acts as a slow-poisoning agent in the person who fails to bear the burden of workload and/or the mental strain.

Stress as a phenomenon increases with the rapid industrialization in this techno-commercio-managerial age. As more and more mechanization is relieving humans from the orgy of human labour, the load on the mind and psyche increases. Robots taking the load in the mine, furnace and poison chambers are de-channelizing streams of psychosomatic load in the mind of humans. The usual reasons of stress impact through the externals upon the human mind.

Stress Management through Indian Insight   **25**

Stress is a kind of perceived pressure, and in the organizational context, usually, it involves workload, both in quality and in magnitude. On the other hand, in the individual context, stress may be felt from other areas of interactions, such as the family, society and environment at large. While stress is embarrassing, it is considered healthy under a balanced condition. Healthy stress refers to the positive aspect of the load, whereas unhealthy stress refers to the negative aspects. We can understand that in all situations—the organizations, family and society— stress is not a derogatory term altogether; it has positive uses for individuals as well as society.

This section discusses the relationship between

1. Stress and quality of life
2. Organizational stress and individual stress

The approach used in this section may be considered as the system approach based on Indian insights.

STRESS: THE NEED FOR ITS MANAGEMENT

Eve Warren and Caroline Toll have explained the stress tightropes:

1. A demand made on us
2. Constraints that limit our capacity to meet the demand made seem greater
3. Available supports help us to meet or manage the demand
4. The effect on us is stress

This description utilizes three parameters—demands, constraints and supports. A look into this matter from another angle seems to be very relevant here before placing our own ideas. Pestonjee's concept of stress audit (Pestonjee and Muncherji 1992) explains organizational stress as follows: 'a situation wherein job-related factors interact in such a way that the worker experiences a disruption in his or her psychological and/or physiological conditions so that he is forced to deviate from normal functioning'.

In their study of computer-related stress, Nebeker and Tatum (1993) have supported the earlier view. They say: 'The pattern of findings of satisfaction and stress may indicate that workers become frustrated and demoralized when standards or rewards are high.'

Before commenting on these definitions, let us discuss the subjectivity of stress.

Stress is not necessarily an external factor and finds the collaborative hand from within. An individual perceives the demand made on him or her in the context of constraints and supports. We may extend the idea up to the area of an individual's inner subjective. Indian ethos advocates that subjective is the cause, objective is the effects, and the quality and expanses of output by an individual depend mostly upon the quality and vastness of the inner subjective of the individual. Stress is ultimately felt by the individual. The degree of feeling of stress by an individual depends upon the inner autonomy of the person exposed to stress.

The cases of the railway booking counter blasts and Jane's sexual harassment as given in the previous chapter show that a greater degree of internal strength could have reduced the impact of a stressful environment. Stress may have its cause in the outside environment, but the individual's response to this depends upon the degree of inner autonomy or the essence of personality. Coming back to the definitions mentioned earlier, we say that stress is not merely the effect on individuals of the demands, constraints and supports but something more than this. Expansion of job horizon and increased workload or the pricking of thorns of events contributes to the degree of stress in a situation but contributes very little (even if reversed) to the management of stress. We shall now specify our hypothesis in explicit terms and try to establish the same in the sections that follow.

The Hypothesis

Stress management does not mean the mere removal of stressors from life scenarios but involves rigorously the entity of the individual. Management of the psychosomatic self of the individual that stands as the management of stress at the unit level and a chain of all these units contribute to the calm and composite fabrication of the environment, where stress is also evident and its management is needed.

In other words, the human personality can develop its capability to absorb higher degrees of stress by elevating its capacity to react to external stimuli. A calm and composed personality who has withdrawn themselves from the dominant trends of rapid exteriorization can cope with the situations of stress better than a personality who is exteriorized or turbulent. The inner subjective of a person becomes more important than other factors. The same situation prevailing in the environment creates reactions of varying degrees and nature.

Our hypothesis aims at managing stress through two ways:

1. By adopting a systematic well-tested and balanced method to develop inner autonomy and poise in a personality
2. By adopting measures to correct the physical environments around (both living and inert)

The Need for This Approach

While most of the studies in the management of stress lay emphasis on the physical fitness of the individual encountering stress and some corrections on the environment that stands as a stressor or the direct agent of creating unhealthy stress, very little focus has been given to the inner subjective of a person for that stressor. The human mind can become the best centre for this activity on stress management. Extra-intelligent faculties of mind that can relate to the storehouse of the elan vital of a human personality should be taken into account first. Through sustained efforts of removing the impurities of the mind, the calmness can be attained.

We shall give an elaborative account of the process of purifying the mind as a step to reach the state of poise and calmness. In the process, we will see how the virtual potential of a personality can be roused to a level of active tranquillity and broaden the capacity of people enormously to contain stress either in the personal sector or in the areas of organizational interactions.

We shall now analyse the effects of stress and the major stressors that create stress in a situation.

Effects of Stress

In the organizational context, the most prominent effect of stress is related to work output, business goals and erosion of healthy transactions. Stress acts as a major player in eroding the effectiveness of the organization; therefore, the effect becomes visible in multiple ways depending upon the nature and scope of the business, organizational culture and the management policies relating to ethics and values. The company may suffer a loss of contracts, fail to meet the targets and may be outcompeted by others. Customer complaints may increase, and teams may feel discord. Centrifugality in all areas may be a dominant feature.

T. Cox has grouped the consequences of stress into five categories: subjective effects, behavioural effects, cognitive effects, physiological effects and organizational effects. The attributes of the consequences of stress as mentioned by T. Cox are summarized by Dyer, Dames and Giabque as follows:

Subjective effects: Anxiety, aggression, apathy, boredom, depression, fatigue, frustration, guilds and shame, irritability and bad temper, moodiness, low self-esteem, threat tension, nervousness and loneliness

Behavioural effects: Accident proneness, drug use, emotional outbursts, excessive eating or loss of appetite, excessive drinking and smoking, excitability, impulsive behaviour impaired speech, nervous laughter, restlessness and trembling

Cognitive effects: Inability to make decisions and concentrate, frequent forgetfulness, hypersensitivity to criticism and mental blocks are important factors leading to the behavioural effects of stress

Physiological effects: Increased blood and urine catecholamines and corticosteroids, increased blood glucose levels, increased heart rate and blood pressure, dryness of the mouth sweating, dilation of the pupils, difficulty in breathing, hot and cold spells, lump in the throat and numbness and tingling in part of the limbs.

Organizational effects: Absenteeism, poor industrial relations and poor productivity, high accident and labour turnover rates, poor organizational climate, antagonism at work and job dissatisfaction

This list of symptomatic effects shows that the effect of stress on the individual could be considered a cause that ultimately affects the organisation. The environment prevailed in the organization is also an important stressor. Subjective effects of stress are person-specific behavioural effects, cognitive effects and physiological effects. In the psychological system, the effect of stress goes deeper through the endocrine systems and the nervous system. Both of these lead the stress message to the heart, and ultimately, the human cardiovascular system develops disorder often leading to death. Endocrine glands are very sensitive to external stimuli; they adjust the degree and level of secretions in response to these stimuli. The nervous system, central and peripheral, respond promptly to these stimuli. The effects ultimately come heavily on the life force of the individual. The direct impact left by this interaction is the rupture in the work environment and demotivation of the employee. Persons with stress may easily be provoked to anger and may become uncooperative.

Symptoms developed by a stressed person may be revealing. According to the authors of the Harvard casebook (Mathews et al. 1991), the direct symptoms are emotional instability, Feelings of inability to cope, uncooperative attitudes, problems with sleep, excessive use of alcohol and or smoking, inability to relax, chronic worry, nervousness and tension, high blood pressure and digestive problems.

It is evident from the abovementioned effects of stress and symptoms that stress is a function of the outer environment and the inner disposition. As a source of stress, the environment plays the role of a causative factor, like virus or bacteria which search for breeding grounds in persons, the external stimulus for stress strikes the personalities and finds some grounds somewhere. Techno-industrial civilization contributes to the ambience for creating stressful affairs. Ford (1988) argued,

'The boredom of machine-paced repetitive work (such as on assembly lines) is what most people relate to blue-colour stress. However, even in this type of work there are differences in people and in what they find dissatisfying.' Ford further observed that 'it (stress) is also correlated with poor mental health'.

Some scholars have linked the concept of stress with the classification of self. It has been argued by Indian scholars that the core self is by definition stress-free. Stress is a phenomenon that relates to the empirical lower self, which is the active, blind and surface layer of human personality, while the inactive, witness and the deeper layer forms the stress-free core self. Too much exteriorization relating more and more to the outer self makes us prone to the swaying effects of stress. The human mind which is the control and which reflects centre of the physiodynamics of the human entity relates us to the world; the more we can free the mind from the psychological impurities, the more we can be placed on par in the spirit of the core self. Interaction with the outer world is inevitable in the existential context. Stressful influence of the outer world pounds on the inner world of man. Core self has been explained as the higher one, whereas the empirical face of it is considered lower. The lower or surface self of humans is always hungry, needy and greedy. It is inherently deficit-driven. The higher or inner self, on the other hand, is whole self. It can be argued that the greatest change agents in human history have always functioned from above their petty selfishness and have operated with a broader mindset. It is a question of identity which we are lacking now. We are the real lion cubs but are constantly considering ourselves as young lambs. This wrong identity fragments the real existent and potential personality of an individual. While dealing with the stress factor and its management, we must take into account this factor as the major one to deal with the case. Dyer, Daines and Gialique (1990) place the role of an individual over the role of the system, describing a case of ethics in the operations of Wall Street. They conclude that

> the integrity of the system depends on the integrity of the individuals in the system. Laws, no matter how carefully designed and rigidly enforced, will not of themselves prevent abuses. Playing by the rules of the game requires that individuals and business take ethics seriously.

Rules and laws are always subject to human responses to them. To become better suited to moral and ethical rules, a person must endeavour to discover their real identity. The deficit-driven lower self has the inherent tendency to be prey to external stimuli, whereas the surplus-inspired higher self would remain calm and composed within to be indifferent to erroneous stimuli, better to be a person with a 'giving' mind and remain inspired and active always. John Locke (1959) has put this idea beautifully:

> For, God having, by an inseparable connexion, joined virtue and public happiness together, and made the practice thereof necessary to the preservation of society, and visibly beneficial to all with whom the virtuous man has to do; it is no! wonder that everyone should not only allow, but recommend and magnify those rules to others, from whose observance of them he is sure to reap advantage to himself.

John Locke's view as quoted here hints at man's efforts in spreading the virtues in the society. Our concept goes deeper into the subject and demands a paradigm shift.

Identity of Man: A Paradigm Shift

The most accepted view (predominantly, Western) of a person considers them a psychosomatic animal having a greater identity with the matter. The Indian view of a person is the other way round. The psychosomatic composition of a person is not ignored, but it reveals very little of that person's identity. A person is potentially divine and the moment they feel and realize it, they transcend from the lower sense of existence to the higher realm. Lower instincts in people make them prone to the thorns of outside stimuli. We can make parallels with the diseased condition in people. Sickness due to microbial infection must precede the breakthrough of a microbial attack on the resistance system of the human body. Unless resistance weakens for that moment, a microbe hardly has the chance to get control of the human body. Similarly, as an outside element, stress can get into the body system of an individual. Its basic seat bed is the human mind. Stress finds a seat in the human mind first and then controls the body. The study of Pandit Shambhu Nath proves the primacy of the role of mind over body. Nath (1992) observes that 'mind influences body much more than body influences mind'.

He adds that 'Stress is measured and evaluated in terms of how it is experienced by the person himself.'

Stress acts basically in the psychosomatic cells after gaining ground in the human mind. The traditional methods of managing stress consider man as a psychosomatic animal and deal with the case accordingly. Yogic teachers have more or less views closer to the traditional views. The 3 R model of Pandit Shambu Nath (1992) offers yogic solutions to the problems of stress and suggests rest, recreation and relaxation as the most important tools to managing stress. He wants man to ensure regularity in resting, recreating and relaxing. Only the act of relaxation differs from the traditional views. He considers the essence of stress as material in nature and therefore offers a material solution to that. Shambu Nath's theory is no departure from the other approaches to managing stress, as stated earlier. Managing stress requires a paradigm shift in the view of man. In the next few lines, I am offering a new view of man for this purpose.

In the process of evolution, man is not the ultimate entity but a transitional being. Sri Aurobindo (Satprem 1991) has contributed to mankind a unique treasure of knowledge regarding the evolution of human consciousness. His idea is that in the process of evolution the attainment of the human form is not the end. The transformation of man would take place in the realm of consciousness. From the present level of consciousness (which has many an instinct of animality) man would ascend to the level of divine consciousness. It will be the play of consciousness.

According to Sri Aurobindo (Satprem 1991),

> The emergence of the spirit in a supramental consciousness and a new body, a new race, is a phenomenon as inevitable as the appearance of *homo sapiens* after that of the primates. The only question in truth is to know if this new evolution will come about with or without us.

The evolution of consciousness shall involve the evolution in the patterns of physicochemical processes that take place in our body. We can easily understand the relationship of external stimuli with an inner response. Here, we would prefer to mention the response pattern of the endocrine glands, situated in the centre of the brain, in the throat, above the kidney. The defence mechanism of the body is the autonomic nervous system which aims at balancing the response by responding through the release of auto-immune and related nervous responses. Therefore, stress causes changes in the hormonal balance of the body. A.B. Harris (1979) has rightfully explained this in the following quotation:

> Stress in everyday life is associated with the abnormal activity of the hormone glands. As long as the hormones are being produced in the correct amounts relative to one another, we can withstand much potential stress, but if amounts are disturbed, then our resistance is reduced drastically.

In this proposition, the role of the inner autonomy of man in stress has been highlighted. Micheal Lerner's view of stress is also interesting. In this Theory of Surplus Powerlessness, Lerner (1991) says as under:

> Powerlessness corrupts in a very direct way. It changes, transforms and distorts us. It makes us different from how we would otherwise want to be. We look at our world and our own behaviour, and we tell ourselves that although we really are riot living the lives we want to live, there is nothing we can do about it. We are powerless.

He observes, 'Powerlessness is so pervasive in our experience that it is rarely noticed as such. Rather, it manifests in our experience through what is popularly called stress.' Lerner, a renowned psychotherapist, observes, 'Occupational stress as a major health hazard'.

In his study, Lerner identifies the major causes of stress as related to the physical body and mind of the person. He finds that stress manifests through varied forms in different people: 'It may be expressed as a drinking problem for one and various other problems for others.'

THE QUEST FOR BLISS

A human being is potentially blissful and lives life in the quest for bliss. A human being is desperate in its seeking of happiness and peace. All the gadgets; the technologies; the statecraft; and the social, cultural and other organizations are arrayed in the journey of man for attaining bliss. Happiness and peace are the derivatives of bliss. Right from the moment of birth, a sense of agony haunts a human being and propels them to seek bliss. When a child cries in the birth cushion, they place their demand for comfort and happiness. The mother provides these. The milk feeding makes the child content, who then engages in play. As the child grows up, the sense of agony extends its portals and the demand for bliss completes with this agonizing sense. A human being's realm expands in material content but contracts in blissful content. The educating and training phase helps a human being to unlearn the potent and learn the outer embraces to bliss. Present civilization makes us think of attaining happiness and peace through external means. We are being exteriorized. Our students are made to learn in the name of science and rationality that the achievements that subdue nature, exploit nature and rot the nature are fortune-friendly to man. We are made to learn that making fortune in this present span of life only is our target. We are made to become ego-centric, and this essential egocentrism makes us believe in our rights and claims—what we ought to get and what we deserve. We are not taught what we ought to give or what we do not deserve. We are civilized in the sense that we maintain and abide by civil codes and establish a way of togetherness but with the intrinsic and potent tendency to divide. Happiness is equated to acquiring a lot of things for one individual—a unique position in the organization and society, esteem from the peers and subordinates and the fulfilment of all types of essential or ornamental desires. Even then, we are not happy. The limit of demand and want knows no bounds; it expands unless hit by the similar kind of expanding boundaries of demand and want by the other guy. The obvious result is conflict and war. The demands and wants are at war. Every quantum of demand or warning clashes with a counterpart and ultimately becomes sized. The interaction brings a temporary steady state but helps generate stress in both, whether it is on the horizontal level, that is between people of the same order, or on the vertical plane, that is between people in the hierarchy.

The dominant and motive force remains unearthed to man. It is the quest for bliss that leads man from one moment to the next or from one place to another. Everybody tries to locate and identify their share in the pool of bliss. He translates bliss into comfort and happiness and at the same time identifies bliss and its real nature, man's activity would turn from imposed actions to automatic action. Man identifies his own true self and realigns the relations with the world around him.

BLISS: TRANSCENDENTAL OR OBSESSIVE?

The term 'bliss' used here needs some explanation. It is not the kind of bliss as experienced by Aldous Huxley who used psychedelic chemicals to feel the test of trance or temporary samadhi and remained in bliss for some time. According to Huxley (1980), 'Temporary psychedelic trances through drugs are pitched against samadhic self-realization attained through years of toil for a total and permanent transformation of the whole being.'

The process of transformation as advised by Huxley is obsessive and illusory. It does not help to realize the self; rather, it fragments the scope of the self and leads it to annihilation or destruction. Huxley's type of mind could not catch up with the real spirit. Western scholars have made some efforts but could not reach the nucleus. Descarte's affirmation, 'Cogito, Ergo, Sum -I think therefore 'I am' is ultimately the driving force towards wild ego-centrism and ultra-individualism. We are induced to run after material prosperity in the name of science and rationality. The scholastic view of Bronowski (1951) affirming this, said: 'The insight of science is not different from that of the arts. Science will create natures, I believe, and discover virtues, when it looks into man, when it explores what makes him man and not an animal, and what makes his societies human and not animal packs'. Surely some differences are there. But if the nature and potential of greed, anger, hatred, jealousy and the kind of things are judged in man, then can Bronowski maintain that human habitat is really human in nature? Most probably, scientific rationality is unable to make or remake human nature. It deserves to see the play of bliss if we want to elaborate on his theory. According to the Indian view of man, a person may be explained in five different ways, each of which may be called the *kosha* or sheath. The doctrine of *kosha* (or sheath) as mentioned in the Taittiriya Upanishad (II, 105) includes (Nikhilananda 1979) five *koshas* or sheaths enfolding the soul. From outermost to the innermost, these sheaths are as follows:

Annamaya (the sheath of food)
Pranamaya (the sheath of vital breath)
Manomaya (the sheath of the mind)

Vijnanamaya (the sheath of intellect)

Anandamaya kosha (the sheath of bliss)

The *annamaya kosha* signifies the body or physical covering of man and the natural aspect of individual existence; the *pranamaya kosha* represents the vital or organic side of an individual's existence; the *manomaya kosha* represents conscious life; the *vijnanamaya kosha* represents self-conscious life; and the *anandamaya kosha* is marked by bliss. The aforementioned views enshrined in the Taittiriya Upanishad get types of individuals manifesting the dominance of one or the other type of the sheath—an elaborate exposition of that is presented in the following paragraphs.

Personality types by consciousness are described in detail as under:

Annamaya: Grabbing tendency, dominantly materialistic person who is satisfied only with the physical acquisition of things for the satisfaction of bodily hunger of all types, is an example of *annamaya* type. The person is always the seeker of all types of *anna*.

Pranamaya: *Pranamaya kosha* represents the person with conscious acts of breath. The in-breath (*prana*) is its head; the diffused breath (*vyans*), the right wing; the outbreath (*apana*), the left wing; space, the body (*atman*); the earth, the lower part, the foundation. This type of person is energy-centred. They unleash lots of vital energy for activities.

Manomaya: *Manomaya kosha* represents the person consisting of mind. This personifies the Vedic forms. The Yajur Veda is its head: The Rig Veda, the right side; Sama Veda, the left side; teaching, the body (*atman*); the hymns of the *Atharvans* and *Angirasas*, the lower part, the foundation. This represents a thinking man. This type of person gives more importance to the psychology of action than the action itself.

Vijnanamaya: *Vijnanamaya kosha* represents the person consisting of intellect and understanding. The personal form of *vijnanamaya kosha* is with faith (*sraddha*) as its head; the right (*ritam*), the right side; the true (*satya*), the left side; contemplation(*yoga*), the body (*atman*); might (*mahas*), the lower part, the foundation. This person takes actions based on the advice of conscience and wisdom.

Anandamaya: *Anandamaya kosha* represents the person having bliss. Pleasure (*preya*) is its head; delight (*moda*), the right side; great delight (*pramoda*), the left side; bliss (*ananda*), the body (*atman*); Brahma, the lower part, the foundation. This person has attained the summit of realization and has attained all divinely qualities.

Let us now concentrate on the concept of these five sheaths that have already been mentioned above. *Annamaya* and *pranamaya koshas* justify the character and properties of the lower self, the ordinary man; *vijnanamaya* and *anandamaya koshas* represent the characters of the immanent, the higher self, a divine person; *manomaya kosha* stands as a communique between the two. It helps to link the lower self with the higher, the mundane within the spiritual.

Annamaya kosha is the self that resembles a great extent the need-driven person highlighted by Abraham Maslow in his hierarchy of needs. The person is embraced by the thinking of the essence of food. *Anna* means food and is not merely the kind of food eaten through the mouth only; rather, it means all kinds of foods that satisfy the desires of the organs and the biological activities relating to the existence on the earth. But always, even after the intake to the brim of the containers of desire, the sense of being hungry regains, once again, maybe in another form. This perpetual hunger is the fundamental property of this *annamaya kosha*. It can be accurately termed as the deficit-driven self of the person. Coming to the context of an organization, we can easily visualize that the expectations, demands and felt needs of individuals come from the *annamaya kosha*. The ego spurs from here without considerations of the other. One ego leads itself in a clash with the other counterparts—the result being a gradual disaster on the earth. Too much of seeking, too much of grabbing and too little of giving others lead the earth to the stage of unsustainability.

The theory of the five sheaths hints at the interrelationships among the *koshas*. Figure 2.1 shows the interrelationship among the *koshas*. These five sheaths form a set of concentric circles with *Ananda* at the centre of the circles. The outermost circle represents the gross body, the *annamaya kosha*—the next circles inside are

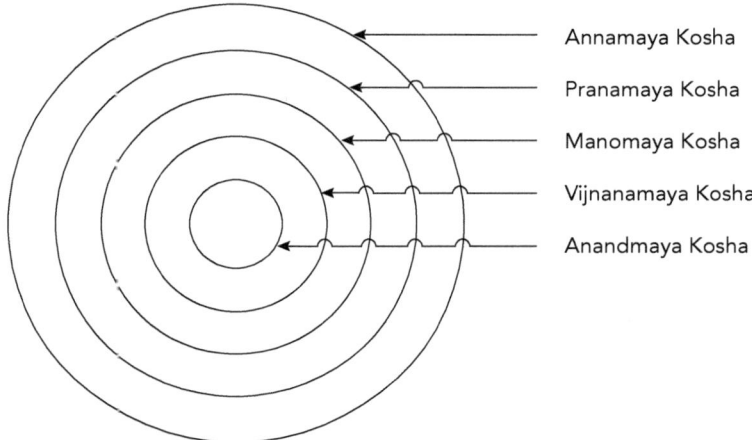

Figure 2.1 Five Sheaths of Existence

pranamaya, manomaya and *vijnanmaya koshas*—while *anandamaya kosha* forms the nucleus of the set of circles.

Personal descriptions of each of the *koshas* reveal their attributes and characters. *Pranamaya kosha* stands on the earth and is composed of the breath signifying it as the stage of the individual when the consideration for the fellow men, the society and the earth system remains very much alive in the thinking and activity of the self. Notwithstanding the impulses that convert man into essentially a consumer, the *pranamaya kosha* finds sense into the broader perspective of life or living humanely. It would not be out of place if we cite a few lines from *Human Values* (Verey 1978), which states, 'It is true that we cannot avoid the concepts of purpose, freedom and responsibility if we are to understand human beings as the essentially subjective creatures they are, or if we are to express any system of specifically human values.'

While dealing with the concepts of the inner nature of man, we can describe this theory of five sheaths as unique. The gross and material outer self gradually converges within. The process of converging is not necessarily one of fulfilling the first step and then passing on to the next step; rather, the stages can coexist. It is a matter of evolution of consciousness from one level to the other. This process is a process of transformation, and it certainly takes the shape of concentric coexisting circles. Rather, if we try to conceptualize concentric closed hemispheres in the place of the circles, we can reach the holistic view of the scheme. The spheres are essentially transparent to the centre. For every person, the very existence relates to the presence of these sheaths, either realized by them or not. The entire zone of activity at each level draws basic impulses from the centre. Few souls have realized the truth of this existence and have come out from the outer shells. Thus, a *pranamaya kosha* may reveal itself coming out of the bindings of the *annamaya kosha*; *manomaya kosha* may reveal itself after being released from the holds of the *pranamaya kosha* and so on. The inherent propensity is always to reach the centre. This propensity is not always identified by the self. The progress or evolution of consciousness tends us towards that *anandmaya kosha*. This progression has been beautifully depicted by Sri Aurobindo authentically, as it was a matter of experience to him. In his words (Satprem 1991):

> A new world is born. At present we are right in the midst of a transitional period in which the two are mingled: the old persists, yet all-powerful, continuing to dominate the ordinary consciousness, and the new one slips in quietly, yet very shy, unobserved to the extent that externally it changes little for the moment.... And yet it works, it grows, till one day it will be sufficiently strong to impose itself visibly.

BLISSLESS IS STRESSED

The ascent of a person to heaven is not the key; rather, their ascent to the new spirit is the task. The evolution of *annamaya* to *anandmaya kosha* would be a fitting journey.

Even if the person resides in the *annamaya kosha* forever, the quest for *anandmaya* or bliss reminds them of an eternal affair, and they try to get a feel of bliss in their realm of *annamaya kosha*. Thus, the desire for peace or happiness comes in the mind of the ordinary gross self. And most of the time, the idea of peace or happiness is translated into material possession or acquisitions. A person may seek happiness in getting well established in the society. They require this much money and that many gadgets to have comfort. They may feel that establishing their superiority over their peers and others would make them happy. Thus, a reward, a promotion, a good work situation or a comfortable pool of command would make them happy. The quest for bliss for them is the quest for happiness. The lower ego builds around it a strong sense of individuality. It is this individuality that wants to be blessed by bliss and that too in an ordinary worldly manner. Peace in the family, peace in the workplace, peace in society and peace in all sorts of interactions become the expectations of the self. The peace-seeker and happiness-seeker find joy in getting peace in a desired manner and quanta, lest the person gets stressed. The root cause of all sorts of stress is the lack of bliss. Bliss makes life enjoyable, comfortable and contained. The person is essentially full of bliss in nature; therefore, any missing link with the inherent bliss would turn them stressful.

The immediate effect of bliss on a person is the joy. Even in a stressed work situation, mental happiness of the worker, the employee makes him work spontaneously. They feel the existence of the sheath of bliss through joy, and it inspires them for their duty. And not only duty, but a joyful person also goes beyond the limits of duty, thereby benefitting and delighting the organization they are into. Spontaneous work has the highest potentiality. If a person can feel joy in their work situation, be it the office, home or the street, they are prompted by the inherent spontaneity that unfolds the potential energy or strength of the person and it is such a situation that leads the person to perform the role of a creator in their scale. Work gets a wider periphery and newer dimensions. No amount of supervision, no quantum of motivators or other usual impulses are required to get the person charged with the work situation. They turn into a self-starter, a self-tuner, and ultimately reach the goal in the most beautiful manner. Happiness and peace enjoyed by a person in these ordinary courses of life differ widely, of course, from the kind of bliss attained by a person through systematic practice of yoga or meditation. A realized soul experiences the uniqueness of bliss and remains perpetually immersed in that. Swami Abhedananda, one of the disciples of Sri Ramakrishna, in his famous lecture on *Panchadasi* (Vedanta) given at the Christo-Theosophical Society at Bloomsbury, London, on 27 October 1896, had explained the nature of happiness experienced by a realized soul (Abhedananda 1967). Abhedananda said:

I have known the Supreme *Atman*, therefore, I am happy, I am enjoying highest bliss.

Th[e]refore I am happy; I am free from the worldly bonds, I am also free from the chain of delusion, therefore, I am happy. I have no obligation to anyone, I have attained the highest object, for which I was practising so long, therefore I am happy. I am enjoying the sublime bliss, therefore, I am the happiest of the happy.

This exposition of Vedanta is highly contradictory with the need hierarchy theory of Abraham Maslow. According to him, the ultimate aim of human beings is self-actualization, which precedes the fulfilment of other needs, namely the need for hunger, thirst, sex, security and esteem. Edward A. Charlesworth and Roland G. Nathan (1987) in their book on stress management have described this need for self-actualization as follows: 'This is the need for self-fulfilment, for realising one's potentials, and for becoming the person one is capable of becoming. As you learn to meet your other needs, strive to find the joy of self-fulfilment.'

Here again, we find the quest for joy. The difference between our view and that of Maslow is that of the divine attributes and animalistic attributes. Abhedananda's discourse on Vedanta hints at this point. The identification of Bliss is immanent and potential in a person, and we must discover this bliss. The Indian Katha Upanishad (Hume 1993) describes the network of relationships between the lower self and the higher self.

Know thou the Soul (*atman*, self) as riding in a chariot, The body as the chariot. Know thou the intellect (*buddhi*) as the chariot-driver, And the mind (*manas*) as the reins or the connecting cords.

This parable of the individual soul in a chariot leaves the option to be taken by the chariot driver to the goal. Goals may differ but the goal of our eternal journey must be the same (expressed or understood)—the passage to eternity and being one with the immutable truth. The Indian view calls it *sat–chit–ananda* (existence–knowledge–bliss). The feeling of the bliss must contain the realizations of existence and knowledge.

Looking from this angle, we find that peace, happiness and pleasure—the derivatives of bliss—can be attained by one's secured journey through the troughs and crests of life towards that truth–knowledge–bliss. An individual's real identity lies here. Every action of human life must follow from here. The essential fallout of this doctrine for this world comes through systematic practices of the realization of this *sat–chit–ananda* in day-to-day life.

PRACTICAL METHODOLOGY FOR TRANSFORMATION

A gradual process of disidentification with the lower instincts and gross material objects helps the inward progression of a man. Disidentifying oneself from the centrifugal tendencies of life and identifying with the interior helps in the realization of the inner self, through a process of introspective analysis, one reaches the state of reality. Indian wisdom offers the concept of *poorna* or the whole through such analysis. Who am I? The answer comes through a series of negatives and finally coming to the realization of the real existence which is *poorna* (the whole).

Concentrating the mind on this self-luminous *poorna* self is the key to realizing the higher self within, the charioteer of Upanishad. Maintaining a disciplined inward-seeking life and regular practice of concentrating upon the *poorna* self through breath control and meditation would take one to that sense. We may suggest certain steps categorically for different kinds of people in the context of modern organizations. Company expectations versus rewards offered during the life of the average manager vis-à-vis the method suggested by us is elaborated in Table 2.1.

For the young managers passing through the turbulence of tension and conflict, the process of disidentification may start with a disciplined approach to meditation. This sort of meditation may be very easy and can be done even on movement. You concentrate the mind upon the charioteer and think of yourself as the self being carried by him in the chariot. This helps to reduce ego and set actions on spontaneity. Gradually, the person learns to concentrate before the *sat–chit–ananda*. The feeling of bliss gradually occupies their mind and makes them more suited to a duty-conscious person than a right-conscious person.

For middle-aged managers who are at the peak of success or achievement, easy meditation and concentration on the flow of the sheath of bliss within would be of help. The posture may be the

Table 2.1 Reward–Reaction–Expectation Matrix for Managers

Manager Category	Company Expectations	Rewards	Employees Reactions
Young managers	Demand, flexibility, mobility and high levels of job involvement	High levels of pay, experience, rapid promotion, a wide range of career prospects	Tension and conflict but high levels of job satisfaction Above-average anxiety scores Considerable satisfaction Some disappointment and reappraisal later on
Middle-aged managers	Continuing job involvement A greater emphasis is placed on performing well in, rather than just mastering, each job	Stability, some steady progress based on past achievement Fewer promotion opportunities	Some adapt and seek satisfaction outside work Others fail to adapt
Other managers	No longer requires total dedication Demands competence rather than contribution	Fewer opportunities for promotion Possibly sideways or even downward job moves	Cannot escape feelings of failure and frustration Above-average anxiety scores

best suited to one, and meditation upon this feeling on the flow of the current of bliss within this invariably leads to the identification with the immanent, higher self and places the person in the organization or society as one full of joy always being a self-motivator at work.

For older managers who are very much anxious about the post-work life and full of frustration, the approach should be total surrender to the higher self. This has to be practised in mind. As one tries to surrender to the higher truth, the eternity takes hold of them and guides them along the right track. They are now transcended to the *anandmaya kosha* and become a self-starter as well as inspirer to others.

In general, for all categories of people, the method of conceptualizing everything in the existence as the derivatives of the *anandmaya kosha* reflects the progression from *annamaya* to the *anandmaya* self. A person identifies the inherent bliss in each of existence. Our quest for peace, pleasure and happiness is, in fact, the quest for the blissful higher self. The best way to prevent stress is whenever we do anything, work in organizations or at home, we offer ourselves to the *anandmaya kosha*. Bliss seeking becomes the prime motive in life. Depending upon the level of attainment and consciousness, bliss, the ultimate objective, is revealed to people in the form of material contentment, desire fulfilment and need satisfaction.

The task in organizational life, therefore, remains to educate men to know their real nature. Work life then turns into a life of blissful existence. 'I work because I find joy in the work, I live on work' this becomes the mood of the person engaged in work. A person becomes self-inspired and a self-starter and tries to cross all boundaries of bondage that makes the work boring. A person with spontaneous joy reshapes the destiny of organizations. Joy, joy and joy make life inherently blissful and potentially *poorna*. This turns out to be the ultimate aim of human civilization.

In Figure 2.2, we have shown how in the stress-free lifeline, A PERSON correlates the work life with the interactions in life (with social or individual agents), and in THEIR pursuit for attaining

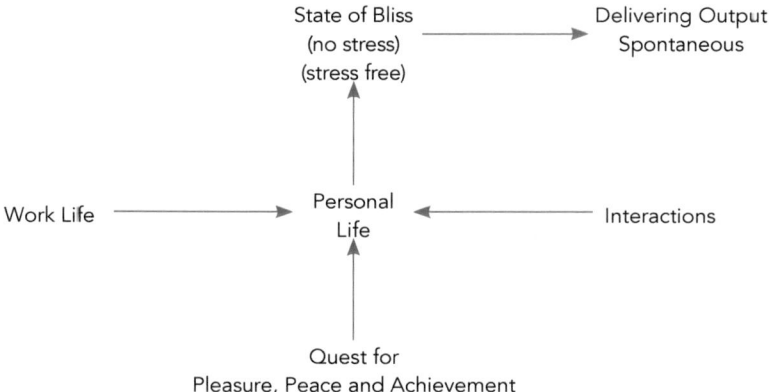

Figure 2.2 Stress-free Lifeline

pleasure, peace and achievements, They attain the state of bliss—the stress-free state. The only spontaneous initiative, energy, output, goal achievement and joy can make this. Work becomes a matter of joy. Boredom and stress disappear from the individual life as well as from the group situations. *Sat–chit–ananda* finds a place in the heart of people in pursuit of bliss and becomes the most formidable tool for stress management.

BIBLIOGRAPHY

Abhedananda, Swami. 1967. *Complete Works*, Vol. II. Calcutta: Ramakrishna Vedanta Math.

Bronowski, J. 1951. *The Common Sense of Science*. London: William Heinemann.

Charlesworth, Edward A., and Ronald G. Nathan. 1987. *Stress Management: A Comprehensive Guide to Wellness*. London: Corgi Books.

Cooper, Cary L., and Judi Marshall. 1978. *Understanding Stress*. London: Macmillan.

Davies, K. 1981. *Human Behaviour at Work: Organisational Behaviour*. New Delhi: Tata McGraw Hill.

Dyer, W. G., R. H. Dainess, and Will Giliaque. 1990. *The Challenge of Management*. San Diego: Hercourt Brace Jovandrich Publishers.

Ford, R. L. 1988. *Work Organisation and Power. Introduction to Industrial Sociology*. Boston: Alhya and Bacon.

Harris, Anthony Barnard. 1979. *Breakpoint: Stress and the Crisis of Modern Living*. London: Thurstone Books.

Hume, Robert Ernest. 1993. *The Thirteen Principal Upanishads* (Translated from Sanskrit). Delhi: Oxford University Press.

Huxley, Aldous. 1980. *Moksha*. London: Chatto and Windus.

Lerner, Michael. 1991. *Surplus Powerlessness*. Atlantic Highlands: Humanities Press International.

Locke, John. 1959. *An Essay Concerning Human Understanding (1690)*. New York: Dover Publications.

Mathews, John B., Kenneth E. Goodpaster, and Laura L. Nash. 1991. *Policies and Persons: A Case Book in Business Ethics*. New York: McGraw Hill.

Nath, Pandit Shambhu. 1992. *Stress Management through Yoga and Meditation*. New Delhi: Sterling Publishers.

Nebeker, Dilbert M., and Charles B. Tatum. 1993. 'The Effect of Computer Monitoring Standards, and Rewards on Work

Performance, Job Satisfaction and Stress'. *Journal of Applied Social Psychology* 23: 7.

Nikhilananda, Swami. 1979. *The Upanishads: Taittiriya and Chhandogya*. New York: Ramakrishna Vivekananda Centre.

Pestonjee, D. M., and Nina Muncherji. 1992. '"Stress Audit" on HRD/OD Intervention'. *Indian Journal of Social Work* 55, no. 2 (April): 133.

Satprem. 1991. *Sri Aurobindo*. Pondicherry: Sri Aurobindo Ashram.

Verey, Godfrey. 1978. *Human Values*. Sussex: The Harvester Press.

Warren, E., and Caroline Toll. 1993. *The Stress Workbook*. London: Nicholas Brealey Publishing.

CHAPTER 3

STRESSLESS MIND
Concepts and Practices

Stress and conflict are normal orders of the day. Most of us are into these orders in some way or the other. People are armed with words, actions or weapons to wage wars and initiate conflict. Even the Lord on the earth also carries arms. The war of Kurukshetra was not just an ordinary war; rather, it was destined to establish the rule of 'dharma' or righteousness in the human society. Lord Rama mentions this point very categorically in the Ramayana with the following words:

Satyena Ayudhyam alabhe
neyam mamamahi saumaya durlabha sagarambara
na hi eeheyam adharmena sakratvam api Lakshmana

(I carry arms for the sake of truth. It is not difficult for me to gain this whole universe but I desire not even the suzerainty of the heavens if it is through unrighteousness.)

The dawn of civilization saw wars and contradictions in the human system that has tended to reset waves of chaos into order. Divine dominance having been countervailed by the demonic avalanches, the process of war did not stop but had changed its pattern only. In a sweeping change of pattern, the modern age has termed the war as competition and tries to contain both sides through a philosophical description of the event as 'laissez-faire'. As Ivan Alexander (1997) puts it: 'If competition were only a form of battle, then victory for one side, and surrender by the other, would mean victory for the monopoly of the victor. It would bring order, but not desirable order.' Such is the case that which makes competition work as a social mechanism is not the pitched battle but the voluntary truce. Competition is a form of compromise. Almost every act in business is a reconciliation of warring probability. Although competition is depicted as a process of reconciliation, it is a war of entities for the possession of resources. The war which Lord Rama initiated was a war determined to establish righteousness. A close look at the Ramayana, the great epic written by sage Valmiki, shows how the process of war was holistically righteous. A glimpse of it is as follows.

RIGHTEOUS ASSERTION

Ravana, the demon king, heard of Sita, a lady of incomparable beauty, and became extremely covetous of possessing her. Sita, the wife of Lord Rama, was living with her consort deep in the forest. Ravana, a demon with the power to change his face and appearance, took the form of a Brahmin, begging alms from the householder. Ravana grabbed the opportunity when Rama and his brother-follower, Lakshmana, were away from home for hunting. While giving alms to a person with the look and appearance of a sage (Ravana, the demon taking that form through illusive, magical power), the pious lady was kidnapped and lifted to the airplane to bring her to his own setting in Lanka (now Sri Lanka) by crossing the Indian Ocean. Demon Ravana did his job like a true demon, while Rama did not reciprocate with a similar strategy to get Sita back.

Hanuman, the great devotee of Rama with more magical but divine power, visited Lanka in order to find Sita. Hanuman could have easily taken her back and return her to his lord.

In fact, Hanuman expressed his intention to take her back, flying through the stratosphere and tropopause crossing the Indian Ocean, back to his lord. But Sita had refused. Her sense of divine dignity wanted the lord to rescue her on his own by waging a war against the unrighteous—not by adopting escape strategies as a reconciliatory compromise, but to confront Ravana and win her. This is why the lord carries arms. Business observes quite a contrasting scenario, asserting the might of Ravana and ridiculing Rama. The result is often quite ridiculous.

THE BUSINESS MIND

Unlike the popular impression, the business develops a kind of mind. The general feature of a business mind is to try and grab things by any means. The motive force is perpetual success which was observed by Whitehead (1993) as a deviation from the mind of the society as 'The motive of success is not enough. It produces a short-sighted world which destroys the sources of its own prosperity. We must not fall into the fallacy—thinking the business world, in abstraction of the community, is largely dominated by the business mind.'

Business mind that creates the ambience for newer social settings leads to changes into newer orders. Is this compatible with the changes? The West's legacy in the Roman system of enjoying the live show of a slave given the opportunity to fight against hungry lions in arenas in his bid to get free is worth citing here. The view of this live fight between a slave and a lion and the obvious devouring of the slave by the lion could yield the maximum charms of enjoyment and release a lot of adrenaline in the entities of the 'civilized' Romans. Do we, the business lords and slave intellect traders, find a fitting heritage in that? Whitehead's observation could be sustained by a few facts.

Fact 1: Obsessive shoppers who risk bankruptcy by buying things of wider choice.

They didn't really want or need many things which were within the list of their obsessive buying. This trend could be saved by a suggestive pill already used to treat other compulsive behaviours. A preliminary study suggests compulsive shopping or buying might affect approximately 1–6 per cent of the American population. According to a doctor, the problem appears to be more common in women, who mostly buy beauty products, clothing, shoes and makeup, than in men, who tend to purchase electronics, gadgets, work tools, vehicles and clothes. Most patients think about buying all the time. They arrange their lives around shopping. But their euphoria in the store is followed by guilt and disgust when they think about what they have done. The urge to shop can be so powerful that people go bankrupt or lose their job because they were too busy shopping to show up on time.

The shopping syndrome was found by many consultants to be reduced by using medicine (Fluvoxamine)—at least to the extent of 50 per cent. The report flashes out a very important aspect of the civilized existence. The purpose is not even being known; we keep on buying. The so-called techno-commercial civilization is based on buying instincts or buying faculties. Unless there is a boom in terms of horizontal and/or vertical usage of products and services, the objective of profit maximization cannot be fulfilled. In the pursuit of enhancing the consumer base and increasing the depth of consumption, the reckless war of advertising and efforts of promotion seldom take care of the real needs but bank on illusory needs. As the report on the obsessive shopping habit suggests, buying takes place irrespective of whether there is a real need or not. Always thinking about buying sometimes turns individuals into patients. The disease being the buying syndrome enhances the worth and bottom lines of the corporation but at the cost of the health of the human mind. What prompted the buyers to follow a course of life to abnormality is a matter of serious concern. Before probing this problem further, let us look into another aspect of the present civilization. This is again the contemporary behaviour of consumers. PTI (1995) reports that a few Chinese were becoming fond of taking the powdered flesh of the human foetus in their morning soup. The report (PTI 1995) says, 'Aborted human foetuses intended for human consumption' are being sold for as little as one pound in the Chinese city of Shenzhen. At private clinics, aborted foetuses could be obtained for between one and 1.75 pounds. Zou Zin, a doctor working at the Lus Hu Clinic in Shenzhen, is reported to have said that the foetuses are 'nutritious' and claimed to have eaten herself in the past six months. She said the best was the firstborn males from the young women. If not eaten, the foetuses would be wasted. A woman doctor from Shenzhen said that the foetuses were even better than placentae in nutritional value. They could make your skin smoother, body stronger and are good for the kidney.

Is this the tragedy or glory of human civilization? The Shenzhen foetus soup is considered to be one of the extreme varieties of the chosen consumable where a human being prefers consuming the flesh and blood of its own species in a nascent form. As cosmic tendency is to maintain a balance, human society now intends to establish a balance through its aggressive habits of consumption—on the one hand, the dominance of physical sex, and on the other hand, the devouring of the nascent offspring. Do we see a trend emerging in the present pattern of consumption? It is obvious that the present pattern of consumption is based on desire. With desire occupying the centre stage of life, individuals try to find ways and means to fulfil it. One desire fulfilled gives rise to another. In the course of fulfilling desire, happiness and satisfaction are continuously being missed by individuals. Desire cannot be satisfied through its servicing. Manu, the great social and behavioural scientist of ancient India, foresaw this problem. According to Manu (11.94):

Na jatu kamah kamanam upabhogena samyati havisa
krishnavartmeva bhuya evabhivardhate

(Desire is never satisfied by the enjoyment of the objects of desire. It grows more and more as does the fire to which fuel is added. Fire of desire is not only kept burning but also flamed thoroughly.)

Desire has been the central focus of human existence. Desire for things required for existence is very much essential. But who is going to measure and put benchmarks on desires? To what extent and not beyond should be the span of desire? Can there be any limiting conditions, any boundary conditions?

It is obvious that corporations, in their pursuit of getting into things, forget about boundary conditions or limiting conditions. Controversies do prevail upon the ideal of corporate governance. Is it just profit maximization or something else? Is profit maximization the goal of corporate existence or the means of corporate progress? These are the various questions frequently asked by the stakeholders of the company.

Corporate progress has been diverted by the goal of profit maximization. In the absence of any kind of softening instrument, the goal of profit maximization culminates in the situation of war in the marketplace. Indiscriminate war in the marketplace could lead to a social situation that is again conducive to a perpetual war of nerves in the human system. Consumption instinct, which has been mentioned earlier, is surely going to induce a fatal kind of war of nerves in society. Direct or indirect consequences are as follows:

1. Breeding conflict, which erodes cooperation
2. Less harmony and more divergence
3. Honour for man is getting replaced by honour for money and position
4. Concern for short term at the cost of long term
5. Soft values of existence being sacrificed to harder objectives
6. Fragmented mind being given overdue credit over the integral mind
7. Noble qualities being subdued for lollypops
8. 'Status consciousness' overwhelming the 'divine consciousness'
9. Worship of the Divine being replaced by worship of money and ego
10. Existential outlooks being reduced to myopic views pushing aside the views of holism

Having invited these consequences, individuals working in organized activities get into work-life stresses more than others who do not

PERILS OF HUMAN HAPPINESS

While walking through a dense forest, a man was chased by a tiger. Somehow they could run through and climb a small banyan tree. The tree was inclined towards a ditch which was by its side and the bed of the ditch was full of weeds inhabited by wild snakes. The poor man, in his effort to be safer, had climbed up one of the branches of the tree which was inclined towards the ditch. But that branch was not able to bear the weight of the man and broke. Because the banyan tree was full of various kinds of weeds, the man did not fall from the tree; his legs got stuck in the thready weeds covering the branch. But the sudden jerk of the branch being broken had alarmed bees that were residing inside the beehive on another branch of the tree. Suddenly, the bees rushed towards the man and bit him thoroughly. The whole incident had alarmed the deadly snakes that were residing inside the bushes on the bed of the ditch. On the other hand, the tiger was waiting on the bank of the ditch in the hope of getting hold of the person, which it considered to be delicious food. The climax of the incident, where the man's feet were tied incidentally naturally to a branch of the tree, hanging upside down, was graced in terms of testing the sweetness of life. From the beehive which was on another branch vertically above the man's trunk, honey started leaking drop by drop from it and as a sort of grace started. This story tells exactly what the human situation is. Surrounded by the elements of destruction, they are absorbing the continuous biting of the bees and thereafter getting satisfaction through the drops of honey even when snakes and tigers are around. What is the future of this person? Can they get out of this trap? Can they come out as an individual free to move and live? Constrained by the conditions, we get enjoyment even though the subtlest of means.

Through its advocated dominance, Alfred Whitehead's 'Business Mind' has created a hell of a problem ridiculing the noble, the gentle, the honest and the truthful. It is against this context that the Lord would like the re-emergence of a new weapon—the weapon of values—to create a value-based system.

THE MODERN RESPONSE

Ivan Alexander believes that the marvels of technology are only wanted if they sustain and promote acceptable values. People continue to cherish old ideals of peace, liberty, fraternity and order. The question is whether the business mind which is creating wider gaps in a global society and more and more sectors of economic as well as social disparity is ethical. A value-based mindset would contribute to value-based management practices in business. The Western world's talking about values and ethics has been the teleological or consequence-driven approach. John Rawl's 'maximin condition' would go to a great extent to protect and enhance justice as a social contract wherein he emphasizes that

1. Each person has an equal right to the most extensive scheme of basic liberties compatible with a similar scheme of liberties for all.
2. Social and economic inequalities should meet two conditions. They are
   a. to the greatest expected benefit of the least advantaged and
   b. attached to offices and positions open to all under conditions of fair opportunity.

Robert Nozick, a critic of John Rawl, supports individual rights in the 'entitlement theory' that he propounded.

While the assertion of rights has been the most generalized view of Western experts, the oriental view has been quite different from this. The Oriental view, particularly that of India, asserts duties of man. Adam Smith's 'invisible hand' tends to correct the market through its macro assertion of considering all aspects of the market as important on varied scales. Potentialities in the market are enhanced through a free flow of various inputs and flow with varied intentions as well as various scales of dynamics. Thus, the market is destined to curb or tame the illogical demand on or expectation of one participant on the other. Through a process of mutual conflict, hegemony and synthesis, the market tends to correct the unethical practices of an operator or a group of operators. According to Adam Smith, the existence of multiple forces is a characteristic of a market, but the process of getting and ordering would be the multiplied assertion of individual selfishness, thereby sensitizing infinite expectation in man. Logical and illogical expectations confront us with a similar set of things and finally getting the result corrected by the market. The basic input for the market would be the utter selfishness of everybody. Maximization of selfish tendency would be instrumental in getting the maximum drive out of the existing potential of individuals

The rule, however, is going to be an orderless order. Gradual fragmentation of the consciousness of the being has been the rule. Both the inter-organizational and intra-organizational contexts are changing rapidly because of the infinite expectation propelled by utter selfishness. Uncertainty has become the order of the day. Even though we do possess lots of tools and techniques to learn the present and study the future, we do not know exactly what could be the situation around to provide for a course of action based on certainties that tend to establish a global society that satisfies the rights and maintains distributive justice. The message for us is to learn how to live with chaos and uncertainty. And not be in the hunch for certainty at a point where it is hardly traceable.

It is going to be a self-doer's society with incipient and emergent uncertainty and chaos. Then, what is the invisible lever that will be holding back and keep running the collective? In a decentralized system as advocated, is it not the collective mind that holds the entities spread out across the boundaries and supra boundaries? Is it not a simple, genuine, honest trust that would be a must to hold the system back against the odds and onslaughts of the disruptive forces?

A sound mind can go a long way to establish genuine trust based on which a future society that could be identified as value-based could emerge. This prompts us to an introspective visit to the realms of the mind.

THE DOMAIN OF MIND

The importance of the mind in human existence has been felt so much that there have been millions of interpretations about the mind. The poets tend to discuss it in one fashion, the scientists in another. Endowing and accepting minds have been the focus of worldly love. A disciplined mind gives rise to one result, an unrestrained mind gives another result. The mind does not stay in one place. Essentially kinetic, it resides now in one place and then a thousand miles away. The mind is shapeless but takes the shape of the object on which it is focused. Intrinsically colourless, the mind can take on the colour of the context of its matter. There has been much research on the mind. It has been accepted as a matter of research by numerous poets and scientists alike. Scientists try to scan it and then correct the irregular mind. The focus of the scientists is to get back a normal mind through the application of various medicines, tools and techniques. There has been much effort to get back a clean and healthy mind, for which a variety of efforts are also undertaken. We should discuss various aspects and dynamics of the mind.

Different States of Mind

In the ancient Hindu psycho-philosophy, a thorough and very rigorous study of the mind was done. Most initiated by the great psycho-philosopher, Patanjali, a series of postulates and explanations of the mind are given. 'Yoga Sutra' of Patanjali mostly deals with the mind. According to Patanjali, the mind has five different stages of development. These are as follows: *Mudha* (inert or dull), *kshipta* (turbulent), *vikshipta* (scattered), *ekagra* (concentrated) and *niruddha* (cessation of mind).

The *Mudha* mind is dull and actionless but fabricates all sorts of ill things. At this stage, the ill thinking of other people occupies the individual. *Mudha* mind does all sorts of low, ill thinking, but cannot translate them into action.

The *kshipta* mind is wild. This type of mind is always in an angry mood- always running helter-skelter. There is no patience. A wild mind nurtures all negative emotions and activates many of them. A wild mind leads to destruction.

The *vikshipta* or scattered mind is always dissipated. It has crossed the harmful stages of *kshipta*, but because it is fully scattered, it cannot focus on things to get the reality unearthed. A scattered mind cannot get peace and happiness. With its characteristic digression, the scattered mind does not help maintain the link between the *atman* and the body. It is not congenial to the unfoldment of an individual's talent or genius. With the scattered mind, an individual loses the fervour and spirit of the inner essence. Unless the scattered mind is disciplined and is made to concentrate, the individual fails to unfold the inner potentialities.

The *ekagra* or concentrated mind is capable of concentrating on one single point. A concentrated mind can help win in life in the truest sense. In a concentrated mind, no ill thought comes, a concentrated mind cultivates only the positive values of life. Noble thoughts reflect in it. A noble thought leads to a noble destiny through a noble act, noble habit, and a noble character. *Majjhim Nikaya* (Buddhist text) has elaborated Patanjali's concept of the theory of cause and effect as follows:

Human destiny is created by human beings only. We reap the fruit of the seeds basically sown by us. A concentrated mind helps unfoldment and sows noble seeds leading to noble destiny

Sow a character, reap a destiny.

Sow a thought, reap an act.

Sow an act, reap a habit.

Sow a habit, reap a character.

Human destiny is created by human beings alone. We reap the fruit of the seeds basically sown by us. A concentrated mind helps unfold and sow noble seeds leading to noble destiny.

The *niruddha* or the cessation of mind talks about a stage where the mind ceases to exist in its present form. Divinity induces at the point where the mind ceases to act and exist in its present form. Divine grace starts flowing in when the concentration of the mind is reached. But this alone is not all. With a new form, a structure, the mind induces divinity and reflects all sorts of divine emotions. Divine grace is the ultimate reward and achievement. Lord Sri Ramakrishna says, 'Bondage and liberation both are there in mind.' The mind that ceases to exist in the usual form liberates individuals. The mind is all. A person visiting many holy places, doing a lot of verbal repentances within his mind and always repeating the name of God but whose mind is engrossed in elements of desire, is not going to receive divine grace. At this point, let us hear Lord Sri Ramakrishna telling the story of two friends (Sri Ramakrishna 1990). The story runs as follows:

Two friends are walking down the road at the weekend. One of them had joined the prayer gathering of a temple where a *swamiji* (a monk) was reciting and explaining Bhagavatam (the story of Lord Krishna). He asked his friend to join the *Bhagavata* gathering, but his friend declined. He had other plans and said, 'Excuse me, I am not a fool to waste my weekend like you by joining the *Bhagavata*, rather I will visit a brothel and enjoy the flesh with all senses'. But after a while, it so happened that the second friend developed a strong sense of disgust in his mind. While involved deeply in enjoyments, his mind was surrendered to the Lord at the *Bhagavata* gathering. The inner man in him started repenting this act of enjoyment vehemently. He felt in his mind, 'Hell this life which is so engrossed in sex and senses. My friend is so great! He is immersed in divine bliss at the *Bhagavata* gathering.' He continued lamenting in mind that if he were like the other friend.

On the other hand, the first friend, seated amongst spiritual aspirants joined the chorus *bhajanam* (prayer song), but his mind was continuously stationed at the house of the sex worker where his friend was. He was thinking in his mind, 'I am a fool, doing all this non-sense of praying to God and listening to Swamiji! My friend is so lucky—he is enjoying the flesh!' The story concludes with the fates of these two friends at the end of their lives. For the person joining the *Bhagavata*, representations of *Yama* the lord of death, had come to punish. On the other hand, to the friend with the empirical body in the house of sex-worker but the mind approaching the lord of *Bhagavata* came the representations of Vishnu. The mind is the central indicator to all. What one is doing and with whom one is working is not important. If the mind is surrendered to the lord and is pure, the person gets liberated and achieves divine realization.

REACHING SUPRAMENTAL CONSCIOUSNESS

Sri Aurobindo has offered a unique concept of supramental. Supramental is divine. Human beings have three states of consciousness: animal, human and divine.

In the animal state of the triad consciousness, a man behaves like an animal. He is prone to jealousy, envy, crookedness, cheating, stealing, anger and lust. He cannot rise above the dictates of his senses. He who takes pleasure in other's sufferings is always agitated in mind. The first three states of mind, namely *mudha, Kshipta* and *vikshipta*, symbolize the animal consciousness. At this stage of understanding, all empirical relations are based on reciprocation. Love becomes an instrument of trade. Arrogance and primacy of 'me' on all affairs become the dominant attribute of this type.

With the evolution of consciousness, one reaches a 'human' state with a concentrated mind, and the appearance of a man then reveals the reality. Man learns to stand and face with dignity and confidence. He continues to be in the empirical activities but ceases to be a slave to sense. His life is then bounded by righteous principles. Qualities like caring, compassion, fellow feeling empathy and honesty are revealed at this stage. He rises above the law of retaliation and reciprocity, which are the dominant attributes of the animal world. 'Human' in consciousness, a person rises above utter selfishness and desire, which leads to the state of divine consciousness.

Divine consciousness is the highest. At this state of being, life is consecrated to the divine. A man does things and gets involved, but the mind is always surrendered to the lotus feet of the divine. Lord Sri Ramakrishna gives the examples of a maidservant taking care of the child in the house of her employer lady. The maidservant does everything for the child, loves the child and gets involved also, but all the time, her mind is focused on her own child whom she has left uncared for. Like this maidservant, we are expected to do everything reasonably required, but the mind is always in the divine world and in the divine's company. This is the state of divine consciousness. At this state of consciousness, a human being is perfectly in unison with the divine. He does work that is based on principles of renunciation of the fruits. A divine person becomes holistic in his view and helps establish a holistic society. A liberated mind or supramental state is the prelude to a holistic view. Holistic management practices are possible only when the leaders and operators cultivate divinity and unearth inner divinity. He is the best manager and leader who has transcended the realms of mind and is one with the divine. Liberated in him, this person can help liberate the myopic selfish paradigms of business management.

Autonomous Mind Is Free from Stressful Impacts

A liberated mind makes the individual great and helps build order in the system. With individuals having been liberated, the collective is influenced and the collective mind emerges out of the bondages of desire.

The free collective mind, being supportive of 'elevated, collective consciousness' helps establish value-based order.

The above analysis shows that a value-based order can be achieved in three steps:

1. Understanding the past and the present properly in the light of the requirements for values
2. Understanding the role of the mind in the whole process
3. Mind engineering for achieving the target of a value-based system

The research findings of the European Science Foundation study on the impact of values edited by Deth and Scarbrough (1995) show a sustained drift in the collective values through changes in the individual values throughout Europe. The researchers have shown that there has been 'an increased emphasis on non-material and emancipatory goals; shifting away from tradition, respect for authority, and material well-being towards self-fulfilment, independence and emancipation'.

The gradual drift of modern man from the process of frag-mentism has to have a culminating convergent. The converging point, however, is not at all any person, a symbol or a system, rather it is a set of attributes that symbolizes divinity. Swami Vivekananda (1995) has squarely dealt with this view in a post-lecture discussion on civilization in America during his famous lecture of 1893.

According to Vivekananda (1995):

Religious thought should be directed at developing man's spiritual side. Science, art, learning and metaphysical search all have their proper functions in life, but if you seek to blend them, you eliminate the spiritual, for instance, from religious altogether.

You Americans worship what? It's the Dollar. In the mad rush for gold, you forget the spiritual until you had become a nation of materialists. Even your preachers and churches are tainted with the all-pervading desire.

Show me one person in the history of your people, who has led the spiritual lives like those whom I can name at home have done.

It is this observation that shows the extent of materialism that has engrossed the mind of the West. The European Foundation study shows the process of a drift from that based on rigid materialism. The above survey of values refers to the progression towards spir-itual values.

According to Banerjee (1997a), 'The ordinary rational mind as well as all human activities are anchored in what could be termed as apparent individuality (to discover the true individuality) the scientific materialistic mind should find ways to have a feel of the divinity within himself.'

The search for true individuality could be done through an engineered mind that finds a role model. Banerjee (1997b) suggests this is the role of a mother. Or precisely, motherhood in individuals. 'Motherhood is the heart of a mother which the country needs so much. Society confronts an emerging situation where the heart of a mother is gradually withering away. We need the motherly heart....'

The need for a motherly heart has been felt by many others, though in a different manner. Vanourek (1995) questions the underlying values system centring on the dollar. He says,

> The management said, 'it's really only the bottom line that counts' makes the dollar its value system. This bottom-line values system does not guide typical daily decisions. If we say it is only the bottom line that counts, what might the shipping clerk do at the end of the quarter when a defective product is noticed? He ships it. Without this value system, what might a vice-president do at the first sign of a business slow-down? He lays off the factory workers without exploring other options first.

The dollar-driven ultra-individualism, according to Adams, will find its way, more profound in nature in the future. Adams (1997) says, The predictable result of the Dilbert principle is that skilled professionals won't put up with the indignity of being managed by idiots. He continues in his prediction saying, 'In the future skilled professionals will leave their corporate jobs and become bosses themselves in ever-increasing numbers.'

The impact of individuality is on certain dimensions of mind, making one envious, boastful of things, of one. A system dominated by self-aggrandizement goes the opposite way in liberating the mind and hence, according to our observation, against a value-based system. The future society can benefit most from mind engineering.

Mind engineering can be based on two approaches:

1. The method of yoga as explained in the chapters that follow.
2. The method of surrender

The Method of Surrender

The same effect, or in many cases far superior effect, could be achieved through surrender. Surrender demands an identified entity of the divine. Once that is done, surrender works out marvels. The idea and outlook being, 'I am insignificant, you are all' and 'Thy Will be done'. A unique example of this is available in the form of Swami Vivekananda. Vivekananda had earned global fame and established his supremacy, but his supremacy was based on a surrender attitude. He used to consider himself as the most insignificant and attributed all successes to his mentor, Lord, in the form of Sri Ramakrishna. Hymns dedicated to Sri Ramakrishna by Swami Vivekananda (1995) runs as follows,

> Om! Hrim! Thou art the true, the imperturbable One,
> transcending three Gunas and yet adored for their virtues!
> In as much as I do not worship day and night, with yearning,
> Thy compassionate lotus feet which destroy all ignorance,
> therefore, O Thou friend to the lowly.
> Thou art my only refuge.

A surrendered mind creates personalities that are humble enough to create a well-cemented collective, the cultivation of collective consciousness. This is perhaps the most dependable way to have a stress-free and value-based order.

BIBLIOGRAPHY

Adams, S. 1997. *The Dilbert Future*. London: Boxtree.

Alexander, I. 1997. *The Civilized Market*. Oxford: Capstone.

Banerjee, R. P. 1997a, January. 'Vivekananda's Concept of Individuality in the Context of Teamwork in Organisation'. Prabuddha Bharata, Centenary of Swami Vivekananda's Return to India.

Banerjee, R. P. 1997b. 'In Search of a Mother: The Missing Motherhood in a Liberalised Economy'. In *Globalisation and Dimensions of Management in India*, edited by Atmanand, 28. New Delhi: Shipra Publications.

Deth, J. W. van, and E. Scarbrough, eds. 1995. *The Impact of Values*. Oxford: Oxford University Press.

Handy, C. 1997. 'Finding Sense of Uncertainty'. In *Rethinking the Future*, edited by R. Gibson. Hachette: Nicholas Brealey Publishing.

PTI. 1995. 'Chinese Eating Aborted Human Features'. *Times of India*, Delhi, 15 April.

Soros, G. 1994. *The Alchemy of Finance: Reading the Mind of the Market*. New York: John Wiley.

Sri Anirvan. 1988. *Inner Yoga*, translated by S. N. Chatterjee. New Delhi: Voice of India.

Sri Ramakrishna. 1990. *Gospel of Sri Ramakrishna*. Calcutta: Advaita Ashrama.

Vanourek, R. A. 1995. 'Servant Leadership and the Future'. In *Reflections on Leadership*, edited by L. C. Spears. New York: John Wiley.

Vivekananda, S. 1995. *The Complete Works*, Vol. 8. Mayavati: Advaita Ashrama.

Whitehead, A. N. 1993. *Adventures of Ideas*. London: Cambridge University Press.

CHAPTER 4

CASE STUDY IN STRESS MANAGEMENT

VICTORY OF THE VIRTUOUS

Sitting in his chamber at the corporate head office at 9 o'clock, the managing director (MD) of a large public enterprise was discussing some important issues with Mr Chandra, the chief internal auditor of the organization. Mr Chandra is placed functionally under the control of the finance division, but by virtue of his posting in the tea division, he is placed administratively under the general manager (GM—tea division). In the corporate hierarchy, functional directors are placed just below the MD and down the line are the ranks of GMs, deputy general managers (DGMs) and senior managers. The chief internal auditor of a division is in the rank of DGM.

MD: I find many interesting points to note and act upon in the audit report you have submitted for the tea division. Irregularities in the functioning of the GM (tea division) as you have shown in the report appear rather surprising to me. But I think I should merit your report, which contains suggestions that inventory of our brand of tea held by the concerned brokers requires to be taken into account by the finance department after proper physical verification of the stock at the end of each year. I think this will protect the interest of the company. Do you have anything else to say over and above this report?

Chandra: Sir, the report happens to be instrumental in inviting so many hard blows from the administrative authority under which I am placed. To be very frank, the GM (tea division) is so biased against me now that he is going to submit an adverse report to you against me. He has expressed his utter dissatisfaction with me and shown anger also. I sincerely believe that people with a sole inclination towards self-interest would jeopardize the fate of the corporation, and I hope you will take suitable remedial steps to save the company from the hands of these people. We should get hold of the stock lying with the broker. I have shown in the audit report submitted by me that situational evidence establishes the particular quantity of stock to be ours.

MD: But how can there be stock of this company lying in the warehouse of the brokers? If you have any additional information to give or any particular explanation of the report to offer, please do that.

Chandra: It indicates that a carriage containing 45 bags of tea were taken out of our main godown in the evening of 30th of March, the day just prior to the date on which annual physical verification of stock took place. You must have seen that the actual physical stock is found at par with that required as per the books of records and registers. Even then I have commented upon the quantum of physical stock to be less than that should have been. This is primarily because tea blending results in quantum appreciation at various proportions of the volume depending upon the components of the blend.

MD: Are you sure about this appreciation in volume?

Chandra: Yes Sir, I am sure about it. It is not a bookish knowledge of mine. I have personally verified this and found it true always. (Discussion with Chandra ends here. Chandra disappears. MD calls Mr Gupta, DGM (tea division) and Mr Sen, GM (Finance) in his chamber in the afternoon).

MD: Gupta, the GM (tea division) is away in Egypt. Now, since you are the man in charge of the tea division, you must explain why 45 bags of tea owned by this company lie outside the premises of the company without any official cognizance. Why did you not mention earlier that a mixture of different types of tea leaves results in higher volume, that is, gain in stock? On what authority you have allowed the additional inventory of tea to be stocked at the broker's godown?

Gupta: Sir, believe me, I do not know all these things. I am one with Mr Chandra in respect of assigning 45 bags of tea as our own stock and regarding other matters, as because my seniors seem to be involved, I find no word of reply to give. (The MD then asks Mr Sen, GM (Finance) to highlight the legal problems if any. But as nothing was expressed by Mr Sen, MD requested him to submit a report to him by end of the day along with his comments on the audit report submitted by Mr Chandra. Mr Sen goes back to his chamber and discusses the issue with some people close to him. After some time, as the group desired him to do so, Mr Sen contacted the GM [tea division] and Director [Finance] who were touring Egypt at that point in time.)

(Chandra's chamber in the afternoon)

Ghosh: Chandra, you have taken a great risk in submitting such a report revealing large-scale corruption. Do you believe GM (tea division) to be the sole culprit or do you see the shadow of other persons superior in a position involved too?

Chandra: Ghosh, among my colleagues, you are my best friend. I can speak to you frankly. People who were instrumental in sending two shipments of damaged tea to Egypt at a lower price have their long hands involved in this case also.

Ghosh: I do not know exactly what happened in that case of shipping damaged tea to Egypt.

Chandra: *A huge quantity of tea got damaged during the 1988's flood in the warehouse of our broker. They were supposed to supply the said consignment of tea to us, but before that, the devastating flood had occurred. The broker could make an arrangement with the GM (tea division) and of course with active support from the* Director (Finance) *managed to supply the same to us at a price slightly lower than the usual level and with the verbal assurance of helping them get an international purchaser. The tender floated by* *the Egyptian government was attended by us offering a price lower than that of the usual market. In this way, they could win the bid. They managed to collect favourable quality certificates from the international inspecting authority. As they found the consignment of tea in damaged condition, bribery took a major role for them to certify the lot. The Egyptian authority allowed the material to be unloaded there for the time being. On quality tests, the entire lot was rejected.* Now, without waiting for the fate of the first consignment of tea exported to Egypt, these people had shipped the balance quantity. This was done probably to clear the central warehouse of our company of the damaged lot of tea to prevent whispers. Again, the second lot was declared fully rejected by the Egyptian authority. At this point, the group could convince the board of the urgent need of their visit to Egypt with the mission to bargain and sell the entire consignment there so that at least the transport costs are met and they can save their face.

Ghosh: But the said deal was finalized by the highest authority of this company, how can we blame only these two persons GM (tea division) and Director (Finance)?

Chandra: Maybe. But these two persons were instrumental in getting the orders passed by the highest authority. (Prompted by the telephonic message from Gupta, GM [tea division], the Director [Finance] came back immediately. GM [tea division] joined the office a few days later and called Chandra in his chamber. The moment Chandra entered the GM's chamber, he was rather surprised to see the glowing face of the former. Without any hesitation, the GM pounced heavily on Chandra with sharp abusive words even uttering the names of Chandra's parents. This scolding lasted for more than 10 minutes. A perplexed Chandra had no option but to come back to his own chamber even without any voice of protest.)

Chandra: (Soliloquy) My God. I wanted to do something better for our organization, but now what is this happening? It is impossible to absorb all these obnoxious words showered on me, even involving the names of my parents. I must quit this organization. I must resign. I cannot work any longer with these corrupt and bad elements. (Chandra writes his resignation letter and submits it to the secretary to the MD and comes back to his seat quietly. After some time, he was summoned by the MD.)

MD: Chandra, what is this resignation for?

Chandra: Sir, it is difficult to work in a situation where the boss pounces heavily with sharp abusive words involving the names of my parents. The honour and gratitude which the parents deserve from their offspring are more important and worthier to me than mere being in a service like this, sacrificing those things. Sorry! I cannot pull myself down to that hell.

MD: With full sympathy to you for your cause, I request you to reconsider your resignation. It is true that being a chartered accountant, it would not be difficult for you to get a job now at this middle age, but my suggestion remains the same. (Chandra refuses once again to withdraw the resignation. Then in a fatherly tone of love, the MD advises Chandra to come to him in case of any vital need in the future. The next day, the managing committee of the company meets to discuss the audit report and the matter of rejection of two consignments of tea by the Egyptian authority. It was decided to dismiss the Director [Finance] and the GM [tea division] from the services of the company and to give an open offer to Mr Chandra for reappointment in the same rank as he had held before leaving the company.)

WORK-LIFE STRESS

In the modern world, stress has been associated with the working condition and nature of work vis-à-vis the coping capacity of the individuals. Problems faced by an individual in their work life do enhance stress and engineer its effect. An extreme variety of this is a calm and still situation where the individual is perfectly at peace with work and work is adequately rewarding and most likely to remain so for a fairly long period. The other extreme variety could be retrenchment from the job and remaining unemployed for the rest period of life. Whereas the first situation is hardly achievable and seldom found in real life, the second one is very common and frequent in the world, particularly among the elite section of the masses who aim at a job placement as the ideal parking slot for life. Unemployment, then, could be considered as a stressor of a very significant proportion. Many scholars have worked on this aspect of stress with respect to individual life. The psychological effects of unemployment and likely unemployment should be considered with great importance. The issue has been correctly put forward by M. Jahoda (as quoted in Cooper, 1990) in the following words:

> If it were found that modern unemployment was psychologically less disturbing now than in the past, one would conclude that the standard of living to which the unemployed were then reduced (subsistence level and do often below) had a greater weight in shaping their experiences than the absence of a job, whfch would emerge as a matter of secondary importance. If, on the other hand, the modem unemployed showed similar psychological disturbances under unquestionably better living conditions than in the past, economic deprivation would count for less and the absence of unemployment for more in explaining their experiences.

In his functional deprivation theory, Jahoda discusses the Freudian concepts of ego. According to Jahoda, a time structure and events to enlarge the social experience are imposed by work. This is a kind of social deprivation and it imposes stress on the human mind. The deprivation theory has, of course, been contradicted by Fryer (quoted in Thomson, 1994), raising the issues of pragmatism, methods and empiricism. Fryer looks inside the individuals and talks about the process within the person. He feels that the individual makes way towards self-determination and autonomy and that behaviour is determined as much from within as from without. There has been a conflict of views between Jahoda and Fryer. Whereas Jahoda underlines individual choice and personal control, Fryer argues that institutions impose things on people which clearly underplays the social identity and independence of people at work. There have been a lot of other aspects to look at this issue and, in fact, a lot of other prevailing views also. Among other models, a very interesting one has been the vitamin theory offered by Mr P. Warr (1987, 51–75). This is the vitamin model and assumes that mental health is identically influenced by the environment as vitamin works on the physical health of individuals.

VITAMIN THEORY OF P. WARR

P. Warr (1987) in his vitamin theory has highlighted the influence of factors towards stressing an individual. He explains:

> The availability of vitamins is very important for physical health up to, but not beyond, a certain level. A low level of intake of vitamin corrects physiological impairment and ill-health but after attainment of specified levels there is no benefit derived from additional quantities. It is suggested that principal environmental features are important to mental health in a similar manner: their absence tends towards an impairment in mental health, but their presence beyond a required level does not hold further benefit. In addition, however, certain vitamins become harmful if used in large quantity. In these infrequent cases the association between increased vitamin intake and health becomes negative after a broad range of moderate quantities. (Warr 1987, 9–10)

The imperative upon this view could be that up to a certain point as also certain categories of external impetus could be treated as stressors. P. Warr lists down certain influencing factors as the basic vitamins for work and sustenance. These are useful but also the causes of stress.

Nine basic work-life vitamins according to Warr (1987) are as follows:

1. Opportunity for intrinsic and extrinsic control (VI)
2. Opportunity for skill use (V2)
3. Externally generated goals (V3)
4. Variety (V4)
5. Environmental clarity (V5)
6. Availability of money (V6)
7. Physical security (V7)
8. Opportunity for interpersonal contact (V8)
9. Valued social position (V9)

Analysis of the Vitamin Theory

The work-life vitamin theory may be considered as very useful and appropriate in the assessment of and causal analysis of work-life stresses. Certain factors lead to stress in their absence, while certain other factors when present in abundance lead to stressful situations. The following matrix tries to offer a detailed idea about the role and extent of importance for each of the nine work-life vitamins, showing the degree of presence or absence of those in causing a stressful condition in work life.

Although the vitamin theory provides a good analysis for work-life stress, it may be regarded as a sort of general remark made on the basis of the observed behaviour of the effects of vitamins on the human body. In the absence of a definite causal relationship

Table 4.1 Matrix Analysis of Warr's Vitamin Theory

Warr's Vitamin	Quantum Intake (Q1)	Causes for Q1	Quantum Intake (Q2)	Causes for Q2
Vitamin (V1)	High	High Stress	Low	Low Stress
V2	High	Low Stress	Low	High Stress
V3	Abundance	High Stress	Absence	No Stress
V4	Wide	Low Stress	Little	Indifferent
V5	More	Low Stress	Less	More Stress
V6	Plenty	High Stress	Scarce	High Stress
V7	Tight	Low Stress	Relax	High Stress
V8	Good	No Stress	Low Stress	Low Stress
V9	High	No Stress	Low	High Stress

between the degrees of stress as an effect of the stressors, the vitamin theory may not be treated as the most ideal sort of thing to define stress. With increased or reduced doses of the inputs, called vitamins, it may be said that the exact relationship with the degree of stress may not be ascertained. With the change in certain extrinsic or environmental factors, the quality of the impacts of the stressors may not remain the same. Sometimes in between the employment and the individual, certain other factors might crop up to change the balance of the situation drastically. This problem is addressed, at least partially, in the Expectancy Valence Theory by Feather. N.T. Feather (1992) argues that:

> Within the framework of expectancy-valency theory a person's actions are related to the expectation that the person holds and subjective values (or valences) that are associated with alternative instrumental actions and their possible outcomes. The subjective values (or values) may be positive or negative, signifying attractive or adverse events or outcomes.... The expectations encompass beliefs about whether a particular action can be performed to some required standard that defines a successful outcome and also beliefs about the various positive and negative consequences that may follow the outcomes. An unemployed person, for example, may have a strong expectation that he or she can perform (i.e., by addressing the question asked at the interview and by presenting self in a favourable light). The unemployed person may also hold the expectation that succeeding at the job interview will have positive consequences, the major one being getting the job.

N. Feather's study is an important indicator towards understanding the causal factors for stress at the individual level. Feather and Davenport (quoted in Angelo, 1981) in their joint study of this revealed an interesting relationship that shows the effects of unemployment being more stressful where the expectations of employment were Feather and Davenport 1981 as quoted in. This particular aspect could be seen as one of the most basic and very vital in understanding the causes and effects of stress. Causes are ubiquitous, but the effect becomes positive or negative depending upon whether there have been attachments to that or not. An intrinsic desire in any event or outcome shapes the event or outcome accordingly. This has been mentioned millennia back by the Indian sage, Manu. According to Manu, desire multiplies from one level, one degree to the other through the satisfaction of the earlier stages. In recent times, the same conclusion has been reached by Feather and Davenport (1981) who found through an empirical study that depressive effect in the unemployed was greatest for those who perceived employment as a valued thing and considered getting a job as highly valuable. This talks about the individual attachment to a job leading to a lot of unwanted problems related to the job. In this world of duality, desires and attachment are rewarded with frustration and rebuffs on their proper fulfilment. Occasions of non-satisfaction or partial satisfaction of these are more frequent than the complete satisfaction of the elements of desire. Partial and non-fulfilments are the situations of stress and the persistence of their effects lead to stress injuries. Motivational factors to works are indicators to the effects of job losses on the psyche. Whereas the visible aspect of work is considered as something that is expressed in financial terms and terms of value creation, other effects are motivational and may not be visible. The unemployed visibly lose the standard of living through not being able to earn at the standard of the employed and through a reduction in the level of their living standards; however, one might be in a position to sustain but at the cost of the charm and cherishes of life. This has been quite a good indicator. The joys in life can be fathomed when both visible tangibles as well as invisible intangibles are satisfied properly. The study carried out by Feather and Bond (1983) is very important with respect to this point.

FEATHER AND BOND ANALYSIS OF WORK STRUCTURE TIME

A study was conducted by Feather and Bond by comparing the structures and purposefulness of works among university graduates. The study showed that the unemployed were less organized and purposeful than the employed in using time. As such the lack of achieving something proves more distressing to the unemployed than the employed. Individual behaviour and cognitions are the functions of the expectations in terms of the valued outcomes of their actions initiated in the course of their network of actions. Feather and Bond supported the findings of Bakke (1993) and O' Brien, K both of which showed the effects of employment on stress. According to Bakke, the unemployed develop distress in comparison with the past work experience, loss of income and reduced personal control over life satisfaction. His theoretical comments are not stated in explicit terms, but it seems that Bakke believed in the presence of two things:

1. Task experiences
2. Money-shaped personalities

Bakke made an important point that personal control in an internalized belief system is one of the most important personality dimensions determined by the tasks performed in work and pleasure. A change in the internal-external control system might create an imbalance for the individual. As the individual is equipped with the knowledge of his accomplishments during employment, a departure from that may upset him and a longer period of exposure to these kinds of things would go a long way to change the dynamics of the system and thereby change the internal disposition of the individual inducing stress in him.

Of course, the effect of unemployment is not always the same. Effects do vary with the individuals getting unemployed. Certain categories would only be prone to severe stress. Certain others through their capability might have resurgence to normalcy. Others including O'Brien, an expert in human biological psychology, have drawn a general understanding which can be mentioned in the following term.

Some of the unemployed did progressively lapse into a permanent state of distress and apathy. They tried to do what they could to (earn their livelihood) obtain jobs and maintain their families within the constraints imposed by little money and poor health.... They experienced stress, boredom, anger and despair. But most were not broken by these experiences.

One of the most important observations of O'Brien was that those who suffered the most stress were the people with prior vulnerability. This could be in both intrinsic and extrinsic terms.

Intrinsic vulnerability: The conditions of defeat and dishonour in mind, assuming every cause to be capable of creating effects. This means a category of people who are always prone to stress through their subjugation to the superior forces in others as visualized by them.

Extrinsic vulnerability: This may be the case with money-shaped personalities. Those who believe that job is essential in maintaining psychological health and who believe that loss of employment is a stressful situation primarily because of the predominance of the job-related stress and their regret for the loss of income, a regular time structure and loss of social acclaim or social status.

At this stage, it is again worth mentioning the point of view of Bakke, who observed that much of the apparent inactivity and negative mood of the unemployed was not a function of job loss alone. It was also a function of past experiences which left people feeling they lacked control of their lives. So it could be said that unemployment just places extra restrictions on people who are already stressed. A negative approach in life catalyses the factors of stress which are already within. This is similar to the method and procedures of the disease forces creeping in individuals.

Individuals are protected through various protective organs, and one of the most important routes to becoming diseased is by helping the disease force creep in through the disposition of the mind and body. Unless a mind, a body develops a defence mechanism of adequate power to wrestle, it gets diseased.

DISEASED WHEN PREDISPOSED

The mechanism of stress works similar to the mechanism of being diseased. Stress develops in work life in the absence of certain factors to which the individual assigns most credentials and fails to achieve or keep pace.

At this point, there is a need to study the things that are assigned most importance in a human context. Schematic presentation of the doer of works in different work contexts and internal assertions explain the relationship the doer establishes in the work situation. Transcendence takes place for the doer when he believes that working in a continuum of work is like being an instrumental entity in that. In the next section, we shall try to show the role of the doer in different situations.

LATENT FUNCTIONS OF WORK

One way to understand work-life stress is to assess how the doer positions themselves in the gamut of work. Work becomes constraining, enjoying and rewarding depending upon the types of relationship the doers develop with work. Doer might position themselves as one in the chain or continuum of work or else might identify themselves as the sole actor.

DOER AS THE ACTOR

The situation has been described in Figures 4.1–4.3. Figure 4.1 shows the work–worker relationship when the doer is the actor. Here, the doer develops a lot of expectations of the work. The doer initiates an action and immediately after that calculates the outcomes of the action. In this situation, the doer has an advantageous position regarding their work. They have got a good command of their work and can get it done the way they think best. The doer is

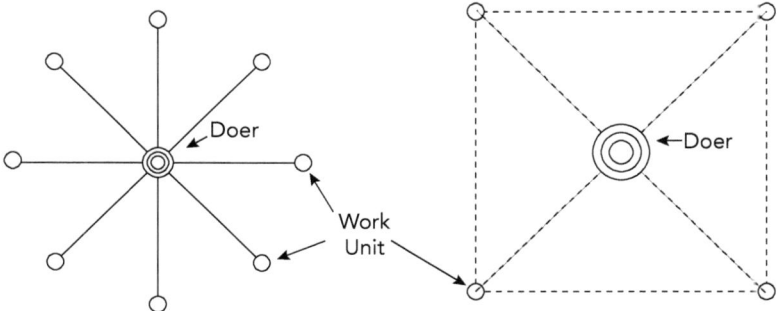

Figure 4.1 Doer as the Actor   Figure 4.2 Doer as the Facilitator

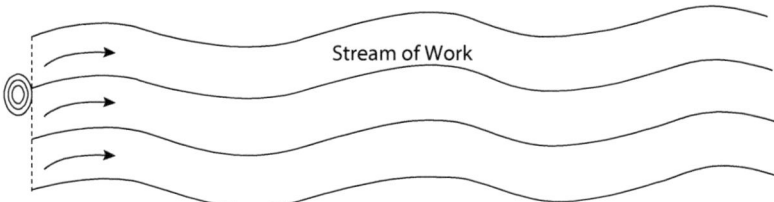

Figure 4.3 The Doer in a Continuum of Work

fully involved in the work as a self and commands fruits designed to satisfy their expectations, concerns and desires. As the doer's selfish entity is involved in this, the doer shall prioritize their self over their role. They will perform more as a person than an entity with the personal desires and considerations fully engrossed in it. Failure in the work then renders as the failure of the person. The doer reduces to insignificance; the doer starts discriminating between what is good for them and what is bad. This situation makes them fully dependent upon the work. Failure to do something means the collapse of the psychological entity. This is well enough a condition to induce stress. The more rigorous the doer is as the actor, the more will be the stress in the likely absence and highest when it is absent; at the same time, prospects for regains are also very feeble. An example of this kind of doer shall help consolidate the view. King Dhritarashtra, the blind king in the epic Mahabharata, is a typical example. Dhritarashtra was physically blind in both eyes, and he was also psychologically blind by being subservient to the wishes of his eldest son, Duryodhana. Duryodhana used to compel the king to accept things of his choice and desire by going against civic and ethical norms. In the king's personality, the father dominated, making Dhritarashtra perform the role of a king predominated by the compels of the father. The role was subordinated by the self, leading to the disastrous end of Mahabharata, with a complete ruin of the dynasty.

DOER AS A FACILITATOR

Figure 4.2 discusses the case when the *doer works as a facilitator only*. In this case, the doer develops a diagonal relationship with the elements of work. The doer initiates the action which is likely to be multiplied by other available operators through a network of relationships. Work receives an impetus from the doer and subsequently the same is carried to other elements of work who in turn puts in their own effort and complete the work. The doer initiates the game of doing the work but does not get involved. The doer does their share and leaves open the rest. The doer operates as a sincere actor, but not the sole actor. They do not dominate the whole of the work nor do they associate themselves fully in the role of operations as the doer. They find in themselves a sort of distant starter who starts off the things and then observe the process of fulfilment of it. They do not claim the work as their alone and recognizes the spirit and impact of others; thus, work becomes a distant factor to them. An important point here is to understand that the doer not only finds themselves separate from the work but also try to get the work a transformed one in the realm of other activities. So, instead of the work unfulfilled, it is engineered towards a superior height of the assigned work.

When the doer identifies themselves as a facilitator, they suffer from a lesser degree of stress.

THE DOER IN THE CONTINUUM OF WORK

Figure 4.3 describes the situations of *a doer in the continuum of work*. In this paradigm, the doer believes that the work neither belongs to them nor to any entity other than the divine. It is the divine's work that is being accomplished by everybody in their respective manner. Divine's work is a continuum of work where each doer has their own contribution. The contribution is in such a manner that the divine intends them to perform. The doer dissolves their individual identity and performs the role of an instrument in the hand of the divine. The work is neither the result of the doer's intention nor the cause of the doer's being active. The doer is surrendered to the divine and whatever they do is but at the inspiration, urge and control of the divine. The divine wants the doer to do the work, and hence, they are working.

In this last paradigm, the doer is the embodiment of the divine to the extent they are destined to do the work. The divine urges others also to do a similar kind of work for them. The work is in effect monitored, controlled and designed by the divine through the divine's inspirations in different persons. The doer who understands the work in this manner relieves the stigma of selfish ego in the work. They work as a liberated worker and a nonperson. The doer hides themselves automatically from the work, and thereby work is relieved of the passions and attachments of the person in the doer. In the realm of the doer, it is desired to achieve a total fulfilment in accomplishing the work. The doer wants to remain divine's instrument in performing the work, and so, they do not try to impose any of their desire, choices and preferences to that. Preferences in the work are determined only on the basis of the demands and commands of the work. This is why work gets complete fulfilment. The doer here performs an eternal job which is not their selfish fulfilment but the accomplishment of the divine's expectations. A surrendered doer of their like does not have any desire in it, and so, the absence of the work is treated by them as the divine's intention again. The absence of work does not discontent or trouble the doer. The doer does the job based on the hint of divine's intention in it; therefore, lack of context, content and the work itself does not create any reaction in them. Work stress or stress due to the absence of work does not remain there. The doer feels his/her role as a subservient to the divine's accomplishment, not doing anything as a doer and then dictating terms to suit their own will or extracting selfish mileage from that in the process of its accomplishment. The doer, in this case, is totally free from the direct or indirect impacts of the stressors in work or stressful situations for lack of work.

Elaborations on the effects of the doer as the actor based on the research shall prove the points discussed above more eloquently.

DOER AS THE ACTOR

Things that bother a doer of this category are As follows:

1. Work structures time
2. Work providing regularly shared experiences
3. Creativity, mastery and a sense of purpose
4. Work as a source of personal status and identity
5. Work as a source of activity

WORK STRUCTURES TIME

Work shapes and sets the agenda for the doer. The doer performs in a manner that the work demands to be performed. In the process, the work inputs shape the usage pattern of total time by the doer. The doer becomes intrinsically interested in offering the doer a systematic approach to the whole of their available time. A doer and a non-doer fall apart on this point. The doer does the things in such a manner that smoothens their concern for managing the total time. The Feather and Bond study of the usage pattern of time among university graduates shows that a doer and a non-doer work with a wide departure in their approaches to work. The doer's days, weeks and months are structured. Loss of time could disorient the doer. Purposeful activity accomplished by the doer differs from a non-doer. A person differs in their approaches to work when they cease to be in the employment. The doer can think of learning through experience in work.

WORK PROVIDING REGULARLY SHARED EXPERIENCES

Social support theory proposes that regular contact with a larger base of social entities provides wider support for the doer. Although interactions are of varied nature, the doer develops a better capability to cope with stress. The coping power to stress enhances primarily through the doer's mixing up with others and releasing the tensions stored for some reason.

Figure 4.4 describes the conditions of work-life stress. In the absence of the scope to share the agonies and anxieties, workplace

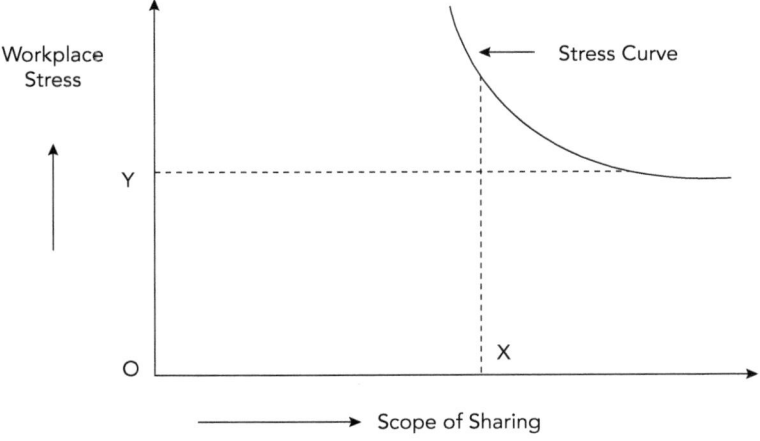

Figure 4.4 Sharing Stress Curve in Workplace

stress may become enormously high, leading to a psychological breakdown. With the increase in the scope to share those things with others, the capability of the doer increases. Sharing of the agonies and anxieties in the course of socializing reduces the burden of stress to a great extent. In the context of the level of stress, the scope to share the grievances, agonies, pains, etc., work-life stress reduces from a very high level to the level of Y. This shows the saving grace of socializing. According to many of the recent sociological studies, social isolation can ease out disturbed mental status in a larger family context than in a nuclear family and also in a larger work environment than in a narrower one. This is the dissipation effect of stored grievance or mental unhappiness. Trower, Bryant, Argyle and Gore support the hypothesis leading to *social support theory*. They surmise that social support from family and friends buffers the major causes of stress and increases coping ability thereby reducing mental illness. Benefits of social support accrue from the friends and sympathizers in the workplace for a work-related stress. As soon as the stress is generated through decay, it is eased out. Decay takes place through sharing with co-workers or associate doers. The remaining effect of the stress remains within coping or managing proportions in most of the cases. The other reason for the increased capability is the possibility of an enhanced level of job satisfaction through contact with more number of people having positive attitudes towards the doer. The doer, being restricted to the job context, is released by the fact that the doer receives a lot of suggestions, examples, metaphors and help and digresses through the increased level of contact with work colleagues and members of the broader community including members of the family and friends.

Through the contacts and sharing, the primary effect could be seen as the sharing of experiences with all those coming into contact. Sharing of experience shapes the course of future work. Shared experience benefits the work in a way that its accomplishment becomes easier, rigorous and more rewarding. Through a support system provided by the social elements around, the doer's problems and mental strain are corrected to a great extent. Doer works as the actor but can get the benefit of diversification. It is like reducing the level of heat content in a metal body by putting it in contact with other metal bodies through a dissipation effect.

CREATIVITY, MASTERY AND A SENSE OF PURPOSE

Work *personified* means carrying on with an individualized tag for the work. This goes against the systems approach adopted these days to do work. In a systems approach, the role of the individual reduces to impersonal contribution towards accomplishment. M. Jahoda while talking about the stressful conditions in unemployment mentions that 'Both the organisation and the product of the work imply the independence of human beings. Take away this daily experience that efforts must be combined, and the unemployed are left with a sense of uselessness and of being left on the scrap heap.'

Jahoda has rightly put forward the hidden agenda in work. An individual develops a sense of mastery or achievement while doing the work. This holds good in cases of satisfying or dissatisfying work. A person occupies a unique position in the chain of offering contributions to society in terms of producing goods or providing services. Through their participation in the social process, they forge a link between the producers or providers and the takers or consumers. Whereas creative activities stimulate people and provide a sense of satisfaction, the repetitive types of work might infuse a sense of boredom. But the creative contribution of the doers helps a lot towards strengthening the mental autonomy of the doer. Work roles are not always important roles. This is very important for professionals and workmen in a competitive and heavily demanding system. In a demanding system, the individual finds no escape for themselves from the context and content of work. So work remains the dominant player for them. It can be stated without doubt that at least for those playing corporate roles, work-related rewards occupy central positions. This shows when someone belonging to the same system is deprived of that, they might develop a feeling of uselessness and lack of purpose. Work-life stress turns into work-deprived stress.

WORK AS A SOURCE OF PERSONAL STATUS AND IDENTITY

A job is an important indicator of a person's standing in the society. Job conditions and positions are important indicators of a person's standing in organizations. Job titles also provide the person a status not only in the organization but also in the society. The person in employment draws esteem from their job title and job position and, in turn, transmits the same to their family. Esteem earned by an employed person through their job position and title is also enjoyed by the family. Thus, a person losing the job loses the esteem also and misses out on the link that they had developed between the family and society. In other words, a sense of losing identity develops. This leads again to a highly stressful situation for the person.

WORK AS A SOURCE OF ACTIVITY

Work is the displacement of a source entity over some time. It is done by spending physical and mental energies and the powers to accomplish work. The activity that is initiated to accomplish something releases the doer from the dullness and depressive conditions of sloth and inactions. Work relieves the individual from fatigue, but at the same time, too much work or excessive activity might again lead to the conditions of fatigue. Repetitive work induces repetitive stress injuries. The mind becomes tuned to one particular variety of work, thereby developing a blurred vision towards other aspects. Individuals develop an inherent tendency to undertake a job that satisfies their various kinds of needs. A particular type of job may prove distasteful after a long period.

A person losing the right to do the work or even losing the expected title and the position develops stress. They lack the possibility of constantly getting stimuli and remaining active. Worklessness takes away the activity and renders the person stressed through fatigue and frustration.

Work-life stress can be more widespread than that have been mentioned above. So far, we have discussed the cases of out-of-work stress. In-work stress sometimes may be even more important and costly. Out-of-work stress fires a shock to the person in terms of the loss of the establishment, esteem and status. It may so happen that loss of work boils down to hunting far better opportunities and making the person more active, more promising, and unearthing the dormant potentialities. In these situations, out-of-work stress becomes less significant. The problem, on the other hand, might be more disturbing in the cases of in-work stress. Moreover, on the job persons become stressed because of not being able to extract the benefits of employment. Employment is expected by many as offering certain benefits to people on the basis of satisfying attributes of one after another. The attributes could be defined as follows:

Job configuration
Skill variety
Task identity
Task significance
Authority
Responsibility
Control

Autonomy

Autonomy in a job context is not perceived as an open-ended-infinite. It is expected to be open-ended but cannot be considered ultimate. To the extent that other people are not disturbed or hurt, autonomy remains an essential attribute of work life. People do not prefer the kinds of work that are repressive or work that constricts or pushes the doer to a reactive and stressful situation. Unnecessary supervision, unnecessary bossing and interfering in other's affairs lead to situations of mental reactions, thereby leading to stress. The degree to which the job provides freedom and offers the discretionary power and the authority to schedule the work is the indicator of the reflections and release of creativity into the work. These days, the demands of the job have changed. Corporations want the employees to be a manager and entrepreneur simultaneously. Whereas managerial acumen is a must for the job, entrepreneurial expertise is required to make the job a success. Autonomy can help unleash creativity in work. Lack of autonomy may prove to be a great stressor.

Job Configuration

Whereas certain types of jobs delight the doer, certain other types are also prevalent which make the job distasteful. Job aversion develops in the kind of situations where the job itself fails to usher in a sense of disliking. Even if the job is highly rewarding, the lack of liking it might lead the job to be stressful.

Skill Variety

Each job has its requirement for a particular variety of skills. The exact level of skill is matched with a job. A job may become more demanding in the course of time, which requires the individual to develop the matching skill. Skill appropriation is a necessity in cases of assigned jobs. Surplus or deficit skill creates problems and might become a causative factor of stress. Skill appropriation is a requirement for stress-free work life. Deviation on either side of the right skill creates stress. Joblessness makes skill redundant so it is prone to stress.

Task Identity

Identifying the extent of the task by the doer is also an important aspect of the work. In-work stress develops in the case of lack of task identity. The accomplisher may complete the job to the fullest extent or may leave it unfinished. The extent up to which the job has been accomplished creates an identity for the doer. The doer develops a particular identity with the work. The absence of this again creates stress

Task Significance

The doer should always be in a position to understand the degree of correlation their job has with others in the same system. The significance of the doer's job to the others is important in understanding the doer's relative position with respect to others. The doer, through this analysis of significance, establishes a network of relationships with people around, thereby creating a work-related society of concerned people. In the absence of employment, the doer feels like a fish out of water with a sense of lost dimension for him. This creates conditions of stress. The doer falls into in-work stress when the significance is either

1. actually feeble or
2. perceived as feeble

If the significance is not felt by others as valid, the doer shall experience their position vulnerable, and their mental world shall then fall prey to the troubles and ripples of the situation, thereby creating a condition of stress for the doer. Even if the task significance is valid but not perceived by others as the same, the doer is looked upon as doing or performing certain tasks that are not relevant to the system and certainly leads to work-life stress for the doer who, in the absence of the task's significance, becomes an irrelevant operator to others in the system. This demeans the position of the doer in the eyes of others who might have expected the doer as having done something relevant to their sustenance and perpetuity. In both the cases of actually feeble and perceived feeble significance, the doer gets stressed.

Authority–Responsibility

Authority and responsibility are the two important elements of work-life satisfaction.

In each task, there is a minimum level of expectation regarding authority and responsibility. Although it is said that authority and responsibility should go hand in hand, in practice, a mismatch occurs most frequently. Figure 4.5 depicts a grid analysis for the authority–responsibility of the doers. This model assumes the following:

1. Authority should go hand in hand with responsibility.
2. There arises a mismatch between authority and responsibility.

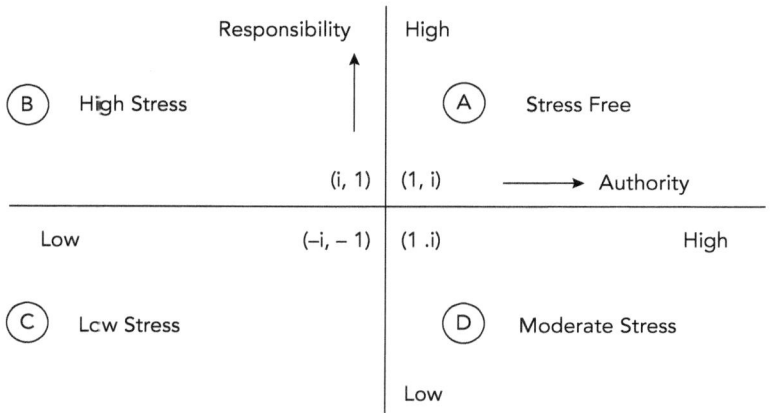

Figure 4.5 Authority–Responsibility Grid for the Doer

3. Minimum or the most desired level of authority and responsibility could be considered as the zero level, while authority and responsibility above the zero level are positive ones till the highest level.

4. Authority–responsibility below the zero level is to be considered negative.

This model offers four extreme types of personalities, namely A, B, C and D. The types offer the following combinations:

Combination A: High authority, high responsibility
Combination B: Low authority, high responsibility
Combination C: Low authority, low responsibility
Combination D: High authority, low responsibility

High Authority–High Responsibility

This induces a high sense of belongingness and identifies the doer to the plight of the organization. An individual, by virtue of their position, commands a good relative position in the society and collective circles. Any deviation in the balance between authority and responsibility disturbs the social acclaim of people. Individuals prefer high authority–high responsibility. Conditions like this are not only demanding but also yielding. Person 'A' becomes stressed in the absence of proper synchronization. At certain point, the person is into a lower level of authority also responsibility. The absolute magnitude of authority–responsibility does not create conditions for stress. Rather, deviations from the balance of authority–responsibility do impart that. Conditions of stress develop when there is imbalance in combination A. A high level of authority without responsibility leads to stress. This happens mostly because of conditions of sustained authority and less or no responsibility. The same is the situation when responsibility becomes higher without matching authority. Performing effectively becomes a problem when an individual is given higher responsibility without the matching authority. This imbalance is again the causative factor for work-life stress. Combination B shows the plight of stressed individuals.

Low Authority–High Responsibility

Low authority and high responsibility breed a higher degree of stress. This leads to a situation when the individual is highly tensed with the whereabouts of high responsibilities which, in the absence of matching authority, is difficult to accomplish. Higher responsibility to perform places a high demand on the person. In the absence of deprivation, one might get into a situation of a level of energy outflow which burdens him physically and mentally. A level that talks about the maximum range of extraction of energy from individuals with or without the corresponding backup of authority. This becomes too sensitive a situation for stress. If along with the lower level of authority, the responsibility is reduced, the problem takes a new shape. It is a condition of low authority and low responsibility.

Low Authority–Low Responsibility

At the lower level of authority–responsibility, it is seen that the individual's attachment to the job is so relaxed that the ego does not develop because of the low levels of both authority and responsibility. Jobs performed in relaxed conditions develop little power to hit back at the person. He can easily distance himself from the job and any minor change in the conditions of work can not hurt the integrity of the person doing the job. The doer then thinks himself dissociated from the job, and he finds a safe shelf for him in the context of the job. Reduced authority and responsibility by themselves are less motivating. This neither satisfies the individual ego nor goes a long way to boost the present level of satisfaction. When one starts at low authority and low responsibility, the worker hardly has full energy and initiative. A sort of negative emotion creeps in for persons with a kind of disillusionment for the job.

High Authority–Low Responsibility

High authority and low responsibility allow a person to enjoy a kind of dominance over others that renders him fit to become the natural leader of the system. A leader without any kind of responsibility is likely to develop stress through the sense of not getting adequate weightage in the entire system. The amount of strain that is present here leads to moderate levels of stress. Job authority absorbs a part of the likely stress in the person. An imbalance is set in the system through high authority and low responsibility. Job title or identification with the job is an important parameter. When a person seems to lack identity, stress starts developing. Although the individual enjoys dominance over the self, they suffer from a dissatisfied ego. The lack of being dedicated is just applying authority over a system without any substantial activity. Without any responsibility to discharge duties, authority becomes meaningless in many cases. Moderate stress that sets in the case as mentioned here is primarily because of the imbalance created.

Control

Control is again a very important factor in the entire gamut of work-life stress. Control has to be at the measured or expected rate and pace. Any amount of control that exceeds a certain limit is going to be costly to the system through the creation of a sort of stressed environment. The other end of control is 'relaxed'. In relaxed conditions, the doer tends to forget about the impact of work-life stress, but they are prone to other varieties of stress, like family-related stress, social stress and personal stress. If the relax condition means a set of indolence for the person, it goes a long way to usher in continuous stress.

In a work context with varying levels of control and motivations for work, the work-life stress changes. Figure 4.6 exhibits the problem with the four different quadrants each explaining its unique conditions of control–motivation and then fixes up the amount of stress that fits into the stage. The first quadrant of the matrix shows a low level of control as well as a low level of work motivation. This leads to indolence. Though an indolent person is rid of the work-life stress, he is prone to personal stress. The causes could be to the following:

1. Frustration
2. Sense of inferiority
3. Relative poverty
4. Loss of social acclaim

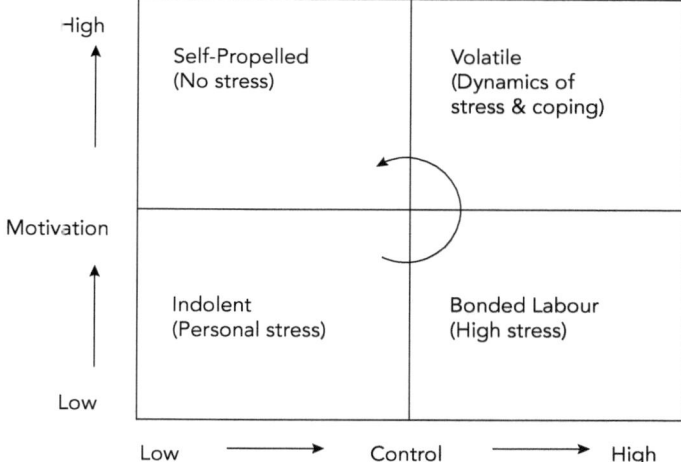

Figure 4.6 Control–Motivation Matrix for Stress

Autonomy in Work May Facilitate Stressless Context

A person might develop a kind of stress which is personal stress because this remains confined at a low level of a control. A relaxed person is subject to the factors noted above.

The second quadrant depicts the situation for high control and low motivation. This is the stage for the highest level of stress. A person at this stage is effectively a bonded labourer. They are not a motivated doer; hence, work is not stimulating nor is it enjoyable to the person. On top of it, since the person is under a high level of control, the mind revolts most aggressively. Work-life stress touches the highest point at this stage.

In the next stage, a person's motivation level is very high and so is the control factor. In the context of high motivation and high control, the person falls into a volatile situation. Here, stress might appear at a moderate rate and is coupled with the coping capacity of the person. The context becomes volatile with high control thrusting upon the motivational factors. In such a volatile condition, stress becomes heavier. In the dynamics of control–motivation as well as stress-coping, people feel like doing the thing; a person becomes stressed that moment and gets relieved the next moment

Case Study in Stress Management

The last quadrant given in Figure 4.6 shows the condition of stress-free work life. Job context that imposes the least control but is imbibed with the high level of motivation leads to a situation of no stress. A highly motivated person, as he is with the least restriction through external control, enjoys autonomy and freedom in the workplace. Work turns into a joyful thing, an illuminating thing for the doer.

If we discuss the basics of stress then the problem and its probable solution will be more clear. As it is widely known, the word 'stress' is derived from the Latin word *stringere*, meaning to draw tight. Work-life stress proves costly to the organization, and its removal is very important in corporate and global contexts.

Arnold (1995) states that 'nearly 10 per cent of the UK's GNP is lost each year due to job generated stress in the form of sickness, absence, high labour turnover, lost productive value, increased recruitment and selection costs, and medical expenses.'

This highlights the gravity and importance of work-life stress in the gamut of corporate work life. Job discrimination is one of the most important aspects of work life. In the framework of Warr's postulate, jobs have been classified into good and bad ones. Good jobs along with bad jobs have been analysed on the basis of nine factors that include money, job variety, goal traction, decision latitude, skill use/development and psychological position. Jobs have been identified as good and bad depending upon the magnitude of these factors. Some factors which are more present qualify the job as good; some other factors qualify the job as bad being in lower proportion. It cannot be said that good jobs are always stress-free and bad jobs are always stressful. Sometimes it may so happen that a job becomes stressful through an imbalance of one factor where that factor had led to good or bad jobs.

An analysis of the attributes as to how they become stressful would help understand the scope and purview of the job discriminators. Analysis of the above given P. Warr's model of job discrimination shows the job qualities vis-à-vis the factors of discrimination. Discrimination always breeds dissatisfaction. Any kind of discrimination is then a likely stressor. In the workplace, job discriminators are not always considered to be stressors. Stressing factors may result in less stress in certain cases. Many researchers also studied the implications of various kinds of the effects of job discriminators on work-life stress. Work-life stress through job discrimination can be more important than the stresses arising out of joblessness, and stress due to job discrimination could be fundamental in situations of multiple stressors. The following analysis should clarify the point here to decide on the elements of stress.

Table 4.2 Analysis of P. Warr's Factors for Job discriminators

Factor	Becomes Stressing When	Job Quality
Money	More than adequate because of security concerns Less than adequate because of the sense of deprivation	Good Bad
Variety	More variety leads to good health in the job, subject to certain upper limits which is subjectively perceived by the person; too much variety poses problems of control and are stressors	Good
Goal action	Inadequate	Bad
Decision latitude	Condensed	Bad
Skill use/development	The pace of skill development is less. This leads to career stagnation	Bad
Psychological	Less in magnitude and frequency.	Good
Threat	But at zero levels, it can again be stressing through contentious fatigue.	Good
Security	The security level is low. But a very high level of security also causes stress through a sense of complete relaxation	Bad Good
Interpersonal contact	Low level of Interpersonal contacts. A very high level of interpersonal contact may lead to a possible breakdown of the schemes and designs of the person for his works which may become stressful.	Bad Good
Valued social position	Less valued position. Valued social position may lead to stress. This is because of the spurious effects of the expectations of social position	Bad Good

Source: Warr (1983).

WORK-LIFE STRESS: THE CASE OF MULTIPLE STRESS

Multiple stressors can have certain positive effects at times. The stressors could originate from the personal, social or organization domain. Studies on the effects of misfortunes on people have shown that in many cases, the coping ability of people to enhance through the impacts of certain types of disasters. Disasters offer a learning process and equip the person with learned tools to face the subsequent waves of stress. Capability enhances with the person's passing through a series of disasters or major stresses. In the presence of multiple stressors, the effect of one stressor on the individual gets diluted through the presence of others. The individual develops a matching shock-absorbing capacity when they pass through major stressors or disasters. Disaster management is a prerequisite to the situations of or the like of disasters in organizations. The process could be spelled out in the following order:

First, the impulse of stress enhances coping capacity by a matching degree so when the second impulse sets in, the injuries to the human system are the least. This has been explained in detail in the stress cube.

The Stress Cube: Multiple Stressors for a Single Person

Stress cube as shown in Figure 4.7 shows the dynamics of integrity, stress and copability. Work-life stress impacts an individual based on the level of integrity of the person. At the same level of work life, the impacts are not the same on all persons.

Persons who depend more on the externals are subject to a higher degree of impact. Stress injuries are a function of the copability of individuals. The following equation can explain the situation well

$$S = K. e^{it} \qquad (4.1)$$

$$\text{Subject to: } K = f(Sh) \qquad (4.2)$$

where S = index of stress-based injury in work life

K = copability of the individual

i = index of personal integrity

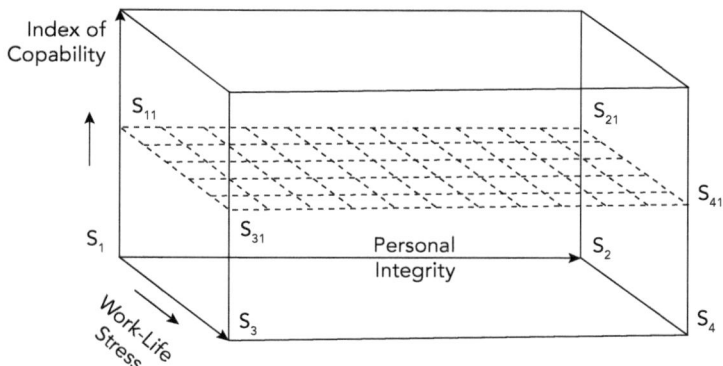

Figure 4.7 Integrity–Stress–Copability Grid: Understanding the Stress Cube in the Context of Work-Life Stress

t = time of exposure

Sh = historical stress

e = exponential base

f = symbol of functional relationship

Equations 4.1 and 4.2 and Figure 4.7 jointly show a complete picture of how multiple stressors work on the individuals in the work context. Equation 4.2 is used to determines the copability. A person's ability to cope with stressors is given here. K is a dynamic factor and changes with the change, in the configuration of the historical stress. Studies on chronic stress and disaster stress have shown a particular type of relationship among the various factors influencing the person. Holmes and Rahe (1967) showed that the process of disaster recovery causes secondary stress. The possible sources of the three types of stressors have been shown as an accumulation of stressful life incidents or events such as changes of residence, job change or change of a particular career path. They also showed the impacts of learning and experiencing in the beginning and then a resultant enhancement of the coping ability of people. In the context of Peruvian earthquake, the impact of physical disaster was attempted to measure by many. Some general excerpts are mentioned in the following sentences. These researchers took two different samples of earthquake disasters as experienced by Peruvians in two cities of Peru: Huarat and Arequipa. Huarat was ravaged by the earthquake, but Arequipa remained unaffected. As both the cities are comparable in demographic standards, Huarat was examined on the control parameters of Arequipa. It was observed that life change units (LCU) rose remarkably high in the earthquake city as compared to that in the control city. LCU as explained by the researchers tries to incorporate the changes in the basic factors of life when an external factor tends to jeopardize the design of the normal life and tends to recast that in a different flow. Other important studies on the Peruvian disaster have shown the same kind of results. LCU's tend to be higher in higher disaster-prone areas and in the post-disaster periods. Life changes units in the pre-disasters or post-disasters varied significantly in almost all the studies. Another study was conducted by Hutchins and Others (1981) on the changes in the LCUs as experienced by the older people in southeastern Kentucky after the area had been severely hit by a devastating flood. The researchers found rapid changes in the social disruption factors as follows:

1. Friends moving away
2. New family conflict

These studies have shown another important aspect of stress that the social disruption factors change so much in the post-disaster period of the disaster-affected people but do not affect the other aspects of LCU's factors.

Friends moving away and a new family conflict are those factors that have natural links to disasters and do change in the process, but other factors such as change in family structure, house shift, job shift and changes in interpersonal relationship contribute to life change in other periods. Hutchins and Norris' study, as mentioned above, suffers from a few limitations like operationalizing the entire effect of the life change in terms of secondary data in an objective manner. Being stressed is subjective and cannot be understood very completely. Life events cannot be expected to measure the stressful impact of every bit of causative factors very completely. There cannot be any continuum of stressing factors. Rather, the stressing pattern and the degree of stress for every bit of discrete stressor event can be caught subjectively by the individual experiencing it. All hassles, strains, pressures and demands contribute to the stressing cycle and continuum of the individual in a continuous manner with discrete additions/dilutions. Further studies on major life events have proved the point that stressing is neither a continuous phenomenon nor a pure, discrete one. It is continuously accumulating through added degrees of the impacts of discrete factors that the stressors direct at. Discrete factors of day-to-day events add to the powers of the stresses coming out of major life events. It has been seen that the major life events impart major learning and enhances the level, scope and degree of tolerance and enduring capacity of the individual. An individual suffers from lesser units of stress with the same type and quantum of inputs. Important research in this regard was carried out by Kanner et al. (1981) who observed that the major life events do affect a person's pattern of daily stressing events. They observed the major events as the mediators to the hassles that might influence the health indicator of the persons through becoming a better predictor of health status. Lazarus and Delongis (1983) predicted the role of major stressors in alleviating a part of the stress, and they observed that as the hassles are of proximal measures, they should be in a position to predict psychological distress which reflects the person's immediate involvement in the social process. They also observed that as major life events are distant factors, the meaning of that may not be the same predictive and influencing all around. Major life events thus have been identified as contributing to psychological distress with more power and rigour than the discrete daily events of hassles, daily stress, individual or collective stressors, personal or work-life stressors of normal magnitude and amplitude. Though the frequency of the major life events is quite less than that of the daily stressors, the amplitude, power and effectiveness of the major events are much more significant and more indicative of continuous stress.

The discussions done above prove the validity of the equation $K = f\,(Sh)$ as shown earlier. With exposures to various major life events may take the proportion of disasters in life. Historical stress (Sh) could be measured by indexing the perceptive level of stress as well as the actual level. Whereas the perceptive level is a subjective judgement of the individual, the actual level can be measured through the study of the direct and indirect measures of it. Whereas the direct impact of stress, as the stress injury suggests, is a tool to estimate the degree of stress, the indirect impact is also an important factor that can be measured again through its impact in a controlled environment. A person passing through the phases of disaster experience develops the copability to combat situations.

STRESSORS LOSE THE POWER TO STRESS THROUGH REPEAT EXPOSURES

Capability

The coping power enhances through repeat exposure of the same stressing incident or the impacts of a major stressor in the life for a fairly long active span of an individual. Davidson and Baum (1986) reported that chronic response is most likely to occur when the stressor of appraisal of threat is also chronic. So, there is a time or relation between them. This study also showed that when stressors rise from the mild stage through an average stage to a chronic level, stress also generates in the same fashion. The stress curve takes an almost linear shape in this condition. Davidson and Baum have explained this sort of linear relationship in their own style. They analysed the case of a technological disaster that was a persistent stressor. They analysed the case of the Three Mile Island Nuclear Generating Station (TMI-2) Nuclear Radiation in 1979 in Dauphin County, Pennsylvania, USA, wherein they found that the residents remained very anxious about the future effect of radiation and felt stressed for a long period. The stress injury, in this case, is acute. A subsequent study by (quoted in Cappione and others, 1997) on the same disaster reported that the radiation effects created a persistent level of irritation among the residents of the island area. The post-disaster factors have turned so acute that people feel the pain in their mind and are afraid of the radiation effect even after a very long period from the incident. Baum et al. view this as a sort of asymmetry in the behaviour, which keeps parity with the nature of stressor-stress curves as shown in Figure 4.7 of this study. These studies prove one important aspect of chronic stress that even disasters that induce no actual material loss may cause lasting symptomatology if the event is perceived as a threat or a danger. Some experts perceived this threat as more important than the material or financial loss. They observed the overall threat and injury to be of a more lost effect than anything else. Lasting psychological distress may arise from damage to property, but the events of disasters concerning life and human assets or a continuous or overarching perception of threat causes more psychological distress in a person. Quarantelli (1985) also affirms this position. This can be affirmed with Equation 4.2 given below:

$$K = f\,(Sh) \qquad (4.2)$$

Now referring back to the equation $K = f\,(Sh)$, we can say that the function of capability is also a linear one. This means historical stress or repeal stress enhances the coping power of the individuals. This condition has been shown in Figure 4.7 as the integrity–stress–copability index as shown earlier in this section.

The stress cube as shown in Figure 4.7 offers a three-dimensional stress analysis. Work-life stress is a factor of the level of integrity of the person, but the effect starts zooming in as soon as the stressors are applied to the individual on a continuous basis. The stress cube offers personal integrity and work-life stress in the base plane and copability grows in the vertical direction through the effect of stress on the person with certain levels of integrity. As the person grows with historical stress, the power to absorb further stress rises to a certain level. The base plane of reference rises from the initial stage of S_1, S_2, S_3, S_4 to S_{11}, S_{21}, S_{31}, S_{41}. This creates a gap along the copability index axis, which can be estimated as $S = 45$ (say). So, one can say that 45 is the amount of stress which fails to injure the person in that context. It can be simply said that the index of coping power the individual has earned through exposure to the perils of stress is 45. In between the two planes of reference S_1, S_2, S_3, and S_{11}, S_{21}, S_{31}, S_{41} the gap created along the copability index, as is the measure of the factor K. Equation 4.2 as shown above operates between S_1, S_2, S_3, S_4 and S_{11}, S_{21}, S_{31}, S_{41}. The original Equation (4.1) is:

$$S = K.\, e^{ft} \qquad (4.3)$$

where e denotes the multiplier effect of the accumulated stress over the original level—which is effectively the K factor.

It operates above the plane of reference shown as S_1, S_2, S_3 and S_4. Equation (4.3) can be explained through the exponential operation of the index of integrity over time. Stress increases exponentially above the plane of reference of S_{11}, S_{21}, S_{31}, S_{41} as shown in Figure 4.7 and as analysed above. Therefore, above this plane of reference, the coping power grows almost horizontally; stress grows exponentially leading to a condition or stage of breakdown for the person. The person loses the power to manage high accumulation and high pace of stress growth at this juncture. Breakdowns occur at points beyond the coping power. A person soon reaches the summit level of coping, and any amount of stress beyond that point leads to the collapse of the person's psychosomatic entity. The exponential stress has not been observed by any of the researchers, but the psychosomatic effects have been considered as real ones in the study of chronic stress. Bolin (1986) in his study showed association of factors like depression, anxiety and somatic complaints with the effects of stress in any situation. Somatic problems are associated with psycho-problems.

The stress cube shows the role of personal integrity and its impact on the process of stress. Coping trends and habits play a significant role in managing stress. A person with higher dependence on the externals is likely to have a higher vulnerability to external pressures and stress. This is very important in the light of the conditions of the surroundings. People with less dependence on the externals are likely to experience a higher level of stress in their work lives. Integrity at the individual level is nothing but an outcome of the autonomy and a state of the mind that helps them to maintain poise in themselves with respect to the externals. Individual integrity is expressed through the qualities of a mother leader. Banerjee (1998) observes that a mother leader takes care of the compulsions and well-being of a person at the personal and the organizational level. Mother leader, themselves an integrated personality, helps others to be so.

The integrity index is a function of the basic qualities of individuals. Although human beings embody different types of values and attributes, the dominance of noble attributes makes them noble. The human state is a composite of different identities including animal, human and divine. The human form can adopt all these different types of qualities. Animal qualities and divine qualities are present in human form. Attributes characterizing these qualities make a man assume animal type, human type or divine type.

Quality Types Attributes

	View of Life
Animal qualities (AQ)	
Arrogance	Kill others for your pleasure, survive as the fittest one
Lust, aggressive desire	
Revengefulness	
Conflicting	
Aggressive sex	
Intolerance	
Irrational behaviour	
Unbounded anger	
Greed, crabbing	
Dominating others, etc.	
Human qualities (HQ)	
Selfishness	Satisfy own hunger
Egoistic	Secure through any means
The primacy of 'me' and 'us'	Cooperate for mutual interest
Anger, desire, sex	
Jealousy	
Envy, Need	
Backbiting	
Covetousness	
Secular attitude to life	
Forming groups according to mutual interest, etc.	
Divine qualities (DQ)	
Selflessness	Surrendered to divine
Sacred attitude to life	Sacrifice
Egolessness	No seeking
The primacy of 'thou'	By the truth
Poise	For the truth
Serenity	Of the truth
Honesty, truthfulness, compassion, caring, cooperation, giving, sacrifice, etc.	

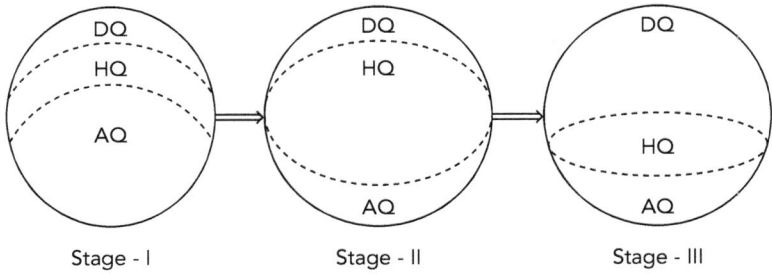

Stage - I   Stage - II   Stage - III

Figure 4.8 Transformation Process in Man

Although human personality is a mix of all these attributes, the dominance of one type makes the personality an 'animal' type, 'human' type or a 'divine' type. Integrity is achieved in the divine type. The human type is the transitory stage of a journey from the animal type to the divine type.

Figure 4.8 depicts different combinations of attributes forming different types of personalities. Stage 1 explains the present state of affairs for most of us wherein the animal qualities play a major role and are dominating in the personality with a glimpse of human and divine qualities in the mix. This man acts and responds basically as an animal in a human form. With some improvement in the qualities in the journey of life, the individual reaches Stage2 as depicted in Figure 4.8. This stage is dominated by the human attributes with some number of divine qualities as well as animal qualities inbuilt in that. The further transition may lead to Stage 3 which is dominantly divine having some amount of animal and human qualities also inbuilt in that.

The dominant set of attributes determines the type of personality, though all the different mixes of qualities are present in everyone. Cultivation of a particular set of attributes leads to an increase in the proportion of that in the personality. This means that decided cultivation of divine attributes makes people oriented to divine qualities and thus makes the other set of attributes take a back seat.

This progression towards the dominant divine type is the journey towards integrity. If a person has the mix of divine qualities, the impact of stress on them is less.

The process of transformation requires a conscious decision for it to be effective and rapid. Dominant animal qualities leave a man in a state where they are highly prone to stress. As they undertake the journey, the proneness to stress reduces at the human state as they grow in integrity. Finally, when they attain the height of divine attributes, they are least influenced by the stressors. An individual who has grown high in integrity maintains life as an autonomous being. This impact of the same set of stressors is very different for these different types of people. A person in the animal state is the worst hit and the one in the divine state is least affected, with the other type at the human state being affected moderately.

The direction of transformation may not be the same for everyone. A deliberate choice is the first step and cultivation of the chosen set of attributes is the next. Cultivation is best possible through a process called mind engineering which has been explained at a later stage of this work.

BIBLIOGRAPHY

Angelo J. K. 1989. 'Predicting Occupational Role Choices after Involuntary Job Loss'. *Journal of Vocational Behavior* 35: 204–218.

Arnold, J., and Bill, J. 1995. *Democracy and criminal justice*, October 1, 1995, Research Article. Available at: https://doi.org/10.1177/026101839501504410

Arthur, Koestler. 1989. *The Ghost in Machine*. Arkana: The Penguin Group.

Bakke, M., S. Kaj, and Tuxen, Anette. 1993. 'Variables Related to Masstter Muscle Function: A Maximum R2 Improvement Analysis'. *European Journal of Oral Sciences,* 101: 159–165.

Banerjee, R.P., 1998. *Mother Leadership*, New Delhi: Wheeler Publishing.

Barkow, J. H., L. Cosmides, and J. Tooby, eds. 1992. *The Adopted Mind: Evolutionary Psychology and the Generation of Culture.* New York: Oxford University Press.

Bolin, R. C., 1986. Disaster Impact and Recovery: A Comparison of Black and White Victim'. *International Journal of Mass Emergencies and Disaster* 4: 35–50.

Cappione, A. J., B. L. French, and G. R. Skuse. 1997. 'APotential Role for N.F1 mRNA Editing in the Pathogenesis of N.F1 Tumors'. *American Journal of Human Genetics* 60: 305.

Cooper, C. L. 1986. 'Job Distress: Recent Research and the Emerging Role of Clinical Occupational Psychologist'. *Bulletin of the British Psychological Society* 39: 325–331.

Cooper, C. L., and R. Payne, eds. 1990. *Causes, Coping and Consequences of Stress of Work*. New York: John Wiley and Sons.

Cox, T. 1978. *Stress*. London: Macmillan Press.

David, Fontana. 1989. *Managing Stress*. London: The British Psychological Society and Routledge.

Davidson, O., and P. Baum. 1996. 'Technologies, Policies and Measures for Mitigating Climate Change. Technical paper, Inter governmental panel on climate change.

Davies, Richard, ed. 1998. *Stress in Social Work*. London: Jessica Kingsley Publishers.

Durant, Will. 1957. *The Story of Philosophy*. New York: Pocket Books.

Easwaran, E., tr. 1987. *The Upanishads*. London: Arkana.

Feather, N. T. 1992. 'Expectancy-Value Theory and Unemployment Effects'. *Journal of Occupational and Organizational Psychology*, 65(4): 315–330.

Gillis, J., J. Tibballs, J. McEniery, J. Heavens, P. Hutchins, H. A. Kilham, and R Henning. 1989. 'Ventilator Dependent Children'. *Medical Journal of Australia* 150: 10–14, 19.

Grinsley, R. 1967. *Existentialist Thought*. Cardiff: University of Wales Press.

Holmes, T. H., and Rahe, R. H. 1967. 'The Social Readjustment Rating Scale'. *Journal of Psychosonatic Research* 11: 213–218.

James, Earnest. 1997. *Psycho-Analysis*. London: Marsfield Reprints.

Jeffrey, Alan Gray. 1991. *The Psychology of Fear and Stress*, 2nd edition. Cambridge: Cambridge University Press.

Kanner, A. D., J. C. Coyne, C. Schaefer, and R. S. Lazarus. 1981. 'Comparison of Two Modes of Stress Measurement: Daily Hassles and Uplifts versus Major Life Events'. *Journal of Behavioral Medicine* 4: 1–39.

Lazarus, R. F., and Anita Delongis. 1983. 'Psychological Stress and Coping in Aging'. *American Psychologist* 38: 245.

Lazarus, R. S. 1971. 'The Concept of Stress and Disease'. In *Society, Stress and Disease*, edited by L. Levi, Vol. 1. London: Oxford University Press.

Marshall, J., and C. L. Cooper. 1979. *Executive under Pressure, A Psychological Study*. London: The Macmillan Press.

McManes, I. C., and P. Richards. 1992. *Psychology in Medicine*. Amsterdam: Butterworth Heinemann.

Nash, Wanda. 1988. *At Ease with Stress: The Approach of Wholeness.* London: Darton, Longman and Todd.

Newton, T. 1995. *Managing Stress, Emotion and Power at Work.* London: SAGE Publications.

Priest, S., and J. Welch. 1998. *Creating a Stress-free Office. Gower Management Workbooks.* Aldershot: Gower Publishing.

Quarantelli, L.E. 1985. 'What Is Disaster? The Need for Clarification in Definition and Conceptualization'. *Research, Disasters and Mental Health*, 41–73.

Robert, Feldman S. 1993. *Understanding Psychology.* New York: McGraw Hill.

Roger, Penrose. 1994. *Shadows of the Mind.* Oxford: Oxford University Press.

Selye, H. 1956. *The Stress of Life.* New York: McGraw Hill.

Sutherland, V. J., and C. L. Cooper. 1993. *Understanding Stress: A Psychological Perspective for Health Professionals.* London: Chapman and Hall.

Thomson, N., M. Murphy, & S. Standing. 1994. *Dealing with Stress.* London: MacMillan.

Thurman H. 1976. *Meditations of the Heart.* Richmond: Friends United Press.

Warr. P. 1987. *Work, Unemployment, Mental Health.* Oxford: Clarendon Press.

WHO. 1984. *Psychological Factors and Health: Monitoring the Psycho-Social Work Environment and Workers' Health.* Geneva: World Health Organization.

Wolf, H. G., and H. Goodwell. 1968. *Stress and Disease*, 2nd edition, Springfield: C. C. Thomas.

CHAPTER 5

OCCUPATIONAL STRESS INJURY

Work-life stress gives us a general picture of the effects of various types of stressors in organizations. The stressors include the following:

1. Role stress
2. Occupational environmental stress
3. Occupational run-out stress

Of these three major aspects of occupational stress, several studies have been conducted in the area of the role of stress. Pareek (1981) carried out a notable study on exposition on role stress and mentioned the following 10 elements that cause occupational stress:

1. Inter-role distance (IRD)
2. Role stagnation (RS)
3. Role expectation conflict (REC)
4. Role erosion (RE)
5. Role overload (RO)
6. Role isolation (RI)
7. Personal inadequacy (PI)
8. Self-role distance (SRD)
9. Role ambiguity (RA)
10. Resource inadequacy (RIn)

Of these factors, the last one, RIn, falls under the occupational–environmental category. Pareek's observation on each of these is explained as follows.

INTER-ROLE DISTANCE

This is the distance or the degree of conflict between and among various roles that an individual undertakes. A person is a manager, a father, a son, a social leader, a philosopher, sometimes all in the same place, in the same person. The demands or pressures of one role naturally differ from the demand and pressure of another role. Performing multiple roles at the same time might prove very costly to the person. Any imbalance or non-fulfilment of the demand of one side leads to stresses on the other side.

ROLE STAGNATION

Getting blocked at one point of the career's journey at a fixed role is a measure of RS. An individual starts discharging one's duties in a role based on certain inputs and with the effect of certain goals to achieve. While performing the role, if one finds that growth cannot be achieved, stress creeps in. Stagnation in the role leads to higher levels of stress if the expectation of progress is higher.

ROLE EXPECTATION CONFLICT

Expectations come from multiple sides and sources. When a person expects to grow in one's career through role changes, the organization, system, boss, peers and subordinates do expect a lot from that person in their respective ways. Satisfied expectations imply the absence of stress, whereas denied or unfulfilled expectations lead to role stress. The higher the deviations from the expectations, the higher the stress is. Role expectations may be subjective as well as objective. Although the deviations on objective expectations do talk about the degree of nonfulfillment of the task, the subjective expectation causes more stress. This is because the subjective expectation is fulfilled and cannot be measured based on subjective parameters. So the attitude of the person or the group towards the doer plays a dominant role in measuring that subjective expectation. Stress, here, is a variable function of the attitude of the assessors.

ROLE EROSION

Roles give certain ranges of powers and positions to the doers. The degree of power and position depends upon the person's feeling of containment regarding the role. Role ingredients are analysed by the doer. An idea or a perception about the RE may be because of certain factors such as perceptive content of the role, actual content of the role and balance between role content and role power.

When the basis of the analysis is the perceptive content of the role, it is the subjective assessment of the gap between the perceptive content and the actual content that leads to stress. When the basis is actual, RE can be measured on objective parameters. Role contents are also measured against role power. Role power is the power associated with a position or a role. Role powers are normally considered as the expected 'shoulds' or 'oughts' of the powers to associate with a role. By any of these standards, the erosion that takes place leads to stress.

ROLE OVERLOAD

RO is normally the outcome of subjective perception of the expectations of a person performing the role. Roles are indicative of the person's outcomes in a role. The roles that the doer performs could be assessed by either a singular standard wherein the persons examine things as appropriate to them or not or in a collective comparison wherein the persons perform the role with the contents in number and magnitude compared to the similar roles in similar organizations or an industry standard. RO is thus the subjective perception of one's doing a job compared to the standard performance of that. Overload means a burden; hence, RO is a role burden which the doer cannot normally accomplish. RO creates occupational injury to the person experiencing RO.

ROLE ISOLATION

RI is the measure of the psychological distance between the role performed by the person and that of other persons. The maximum distance between the minimum role differentials is the RI. Two persons performing the same role in the organization or two persons performing different roles in the same organization may be the measure of RI. This also refers to the distances between the role powers. An example could be given from ministerial roles. Two ministers of the union cabinet may not enjoy the same role power due to their differential closeness to the head of the cabinet. The preferred one normally enjoys more role power than the other. A higher role power creates greater isolation with the other role. In this situation, the lower role power suffers from RI, a particular type of stress.

PERSONAL INADEQUACY

This is a sense of incapacity to perform. PI is a feeling or the actual measure of skill deficiency in a person for the role that he is supposed to perform. A sense of inferiority or a sense of incapability burns inside the person. This type of stress could be personal as well. A feeling of incapacity in family life and social life similar to that in work life is supposed to create stress for the person.

SELF-ROLE DISTANCE

This is the measure of the self's being apart from the role. A person performing the role of a king in a drama is supposed to be one with the role of the said king. This oneness makes the drama rewarding and enjoyable. In practical work life also, occupational roles expect the self to be immersed in that, thereby creating the least extent of SRD. Measuring SRD is again a subjective assessment. The higher the deviation of the self from the role, the higher the stress is.

ROLE AMBIGUITY

Certain roles are not properly defined. If the role is not clearly defined, confusion is likely to arise through the possibilities to perform. RA sometimes leads to a wrong path and a wrong end for the performers, thereby creating a very high degree of stress for him. In some cases, the organizations create and maintain RA with a view to accomplish certain things. Organizations want certain things done based on the role understanding of the doers. Ambiguous roles sometimes do help unleash creativity. But that happens only in a few cases in isolation. In most other cases, they contribute to stress.

RESOURCE INADEQUACY

Inadequate resources lead to a miserable life for the doer. With inadequate or inappropriate resources, it is difficult to perform and accomplish. RIn is one of the most important stressors in government organizations, public sectors and backward organizations. With inadequate resources, job performance is inadequate; thus, the doer makes a lower level of achievement, leading to a higher level of stress. There are certain situations where RIn helps people a lot towards managing through hardship. This enhances the capability of the doer. The doers do feel that a higher level of accomplishment is even possible with lower levels of resources. Inadequacy sometimes creates the idea and determination to run and win in shortfalls, which ultimately helps in crisis management. The work part is well taken, but the psychological distress and continuous sense of deprivation cannot be stopped. In this way, it is always stressing. As has been mentioned in the text before, corporate objectives are now more towards accomplishment with the least number of resources. Therefore, it can be said that RIn is a given condition on which to operate. Higher degree of capability with this helps organizations and the individuals to combat stress.

Occupational stress depends upon other factors like managerial status, the environment in which the person is put to work and other relevant factors. Role stress remains incomplete without the discussion on occupational environmental stress and occupational run-out stress

OCCUPATIONAL ENVIRONMENTAL STRESS

The managerial states of a person become a worrying factor in many cases. Status difference creates worry. According to authors like Boone and Kurtz (1987), there are three basic levels in the management hierarchy, namely top level, middle level and lower level. In each level, managers feel sandwiched by the pressure of the other two levels. Levinson (1973) documented that the middle-level executives find their progress slows down under the pressure of the fresh recruits and also under the impact of the top level. Each level has its unique features and acts as a level with distinctive features. Level pressure operates based on the demands on the level and the ability of the level to discharge its respective responsibilities and obligations based on the abilities of the role. The role of middle-level executives is under pressure from both the top level and the bottom level.

In a broad sense, occupational environmental stress could be spelt out in different categories as stressors from:

1. Physical environment
2. Human environment

Both these stressors are important for the organization.

PHYSICAL ENVIRONMENT

The physical environment has to suit the demand or expectation of the doer. The doer in their pursuit to accomplish may find the physical environment not congenial to their growth; therefore, they may develop disgust and become irritated. A helping and desired environment may induce more output from the doer. The doer's world of work would be a fragmented one with the impact of unfavourable working conditions and the physical setting for the work in an unwanted manner. The external physical environment might prove demotivating at times when they go against the person's expectations.

Some of the common irritants in the physical environment are as follows:

1. Work–home distance
2. Work–home timing mismatch
3. Workplace coordinates
4. Inappropriate leisure timing
5. Inadequate providings
6. Comparative unfavourability
7. Time-pressed targets
8. Abnormal growth targets
9. Work abundance

Doers develop their own mechanisms to overcome the stressful effects of physical environmental factors. An analysis of these effects is worthwhile to understand the mechanism.

Work–Home Distance

Physical factors like the distance of the workplace from home are a worrying subject. Home in the campus of the workplace pleases the person so long as home hours remain unaffected by the pressures of sudden work calls and other occasional and casual demands. Home and workplace far apart mean longer commuting time. Exhaustions in commuting bring the doer's energy level down, sometimes preventing the doers from completing the work in the desired manner. The effect is stress for the doer.

Work–Home Timing Mismatch

Certain jobs demand rotational timing or flexible timing for the doer to perform. The doer might be induced to work in shifts—morning, evening and night. The doer's personal life accepts the flexibility to some extent beyond which there may be some conflict between the pressure on the doer's time both from the family and the workplace. Timing mismatch proves irritating to the doer in many respects and contributes to stress.

Workplace Coordinate

This refers to the site of the doer's work in the workplace. Where the doer is put up and is allowed to perform from the workplace, the coordinate includes the person's chamber in the workplace or the place he operates from. There is always a comparative assessment, particularly among the peers regarding workplace coordinate. A peer member or even a subordinate getting a better sitting slot in the workplace is always irritating to the doer. Similarly, a subordinate getting equal status in the workplace is also irritating. The doer would prefer a slot that brings higher importance to him relative to his peers and subordinates. That he is special should be revealed from the location and site of his workplace. Workplace coordinate is judged from the point of the centre of gravity (CG) of the workplace. If the doer is the head at the workplace, he marks the CG. For others, CG is the radius of each from the head of the workplace at the CG. The higher the radius, the more unimportant the person becomes in the gamut of the organization's operations. Workplace coordinate could be properly assessed through the method of indexing. For a particular level, there could be an identified level of operation for the doer. The doer feels most comfortable in a particular level of work. A doer occupying a work site closer to the CG would feel more satisfied and important than when he is away from the level called the mean level of operation for the doer. The doer is stressed when he is away from the CG and far apart from it.

Inappropriate Leisure Timing

While defining a civilized society, it has been said of a system that allows and fosters

Free thinking
Free thinking for making beautiful things
Leisure

Leisure is an essential component of modern living. Leisure has to be associated with the elements of work. The doer would expect to make full use of the leisure time. The doer has his agenda to use the leisure time. Leisure is considered by many in the literary circle as a good combination of rest and pleasure. It is the right kind of pleasure that the doer looks for. Any other variety of pleasure may not mean pleasure to the doer. In the doer's frame of reference, leisure timing means a proper sense of the thing. Deviations from that mean no pleasure to the doer, resulting in stress related to work life.

Inadequate Providings

Tools required to perform any task have to be there to make the performance a success. The doer has to have the necessary providings to perform and discharge duties. In the framework of the doer, requirements for the providings prove to be a sort of raw materials or inputs to do the work. In the absence of adequate supportive providings, it becomes difficult for the doer to perform. This is another situation of occupation stress.

Comparative Unfavourability

Favours in the workplace play dominant roles in motivating people. Favours are judged on a real-time scale. Every workman compares his position in the workplace in terms of certain factors relative to the centre of power. These factors are as follows:

1. Closeness to the head or the centre of power
2. Identity with the self or the head of the workplace

Workplace unfavourability is highly stressful. On a closeness scale to the head, the workplace favours a closer person than another one who is apart. Unfavourable position in the workplace leads to certain stressful situations. Normally, a doer does not expect any favour. The problem starts when one gets the favour of the head of the workplace. In the absence of anybody getting any favour, things are judged on the merit of the rational demands and expectations of the job. Objective parameters fail when there is a change in the job context through a subjective favour of any person in the system. Stress arises on relative merit to that person's position in the organization.

Time-pressed Targets

In a competitive market and competitive scenario in the organizations, jobs are bound to be time-pressed. Regardless of whether early finish time or late finish time is the standard measure to the completion of a job, when time is a constraint, the measure of stress is the highest. Time-pressed jobs suffer from two types of anxieties:

1. The concern for finishing the job on time
2. The concern for keeping to the desired level of quality for the output

The concern for finishing the job on time is one of the most important worrying factors in job life. Timely completion of job satisfies both the doer and the organization, whereas inability to finish on time leads to a lot of problems including the following:

1. Problems of cost escalation for the job
2. Unfavourable career opportunities for the doer

Whereas the issues of cost escalation bother the organization, the problems of unfavourable career rating bother the person. Both these problems lead to work-life stress. When costs escalate for the organization, the doer may suffer a setback in career progression.

Keeping to the desired level of quality is again an important concern. Time-pressed work runs the risk of not delivering the outputs in the right quality. A job completed within the time frame but not conforming to the desired level of quality may lead to doer's anxiety. Lower quality means more cost burden on the organizations, implying

1. Loss of value for the organization
2. Loss of esteem for the person

Loss of Value

The lower quality output makes the organization suffer from loss of value due to the lower marketability of the products or services. The difference between the original estimated value of the output and the actual value of the same is the measure of loss of value. This loss suffered by the organization hits the doer causing stress in him.

Loss of Goodwill or Reputation

The doer performing at a lower level or contributing an output of lower quality lets himself down. The doer, in his effort to finish the job in crash time, has led to the job output being a lower quality one. This gets an aspersion on the doer ascribing himself for a lower quality output. He is rated as a low-quality operator and loses value in the market or inside the organization. The doer through this timely accomplishment towards inferior quality products hurts his goodwill or reputation, causing worries for the doer. Thus, the situation is highly stressed time-pressed targets, leading to work-life stress from various aspects. Sometimes, it is organization-driven stress.

Abnormal Growth Targets

Authors like French and Caplan (1973), Quinn et al. (1971) and Porter and Lawler (1965) show how aggressive smoking and drinking habits generate high absenteeism and low motivation at work are some of the factors that are stressing outcomes of abnormal work pressure, abnormal growth targets, etc. Abnormal growth targets imply an impossibility to perform and accomplish. Abnormal growth targets are the features of many modern industries. This is particularly evident among growth-oriented industries in developing countries. Abnormal growth targets are the sources of imbalances for many organizations. Certain management styles set abnormal growth targets for junior and middle-level executives. This creates a stressful job environment. The effects of this being

1. A person not being able to fulfil the target
2. The organization being denied its estimated share of profit

Many sales organizations want to make aggressive sales. Abnormal targets may be achievable in the growth sector only by the cash cow companies. Sometimes star companies might adopt a similar strategy with a view to put pressure on the system and getting the highest achievable value. Non-fulfilment of the target does not bother the organization much. The company wants to push up achievements by setting a higher target for the doers. The doer becomes depressed at not being able to fulfil the target. This is peculiar to underdeveloped and developing economies. Sometimes multinational enterprises also adopt this practice as a part of a downsizing strategy

Many companies are seen to grow at a pace of **300-400** times a year. This growth rate talks about a transition for the company from one stage to another. During this transition phase, growth seems to be a must for such companies at those points in time. Transition companies would expect this growth rate as the most desired rate to grow as well as to survive in the market.

In both these cases, chances of faltering and not being able to fulfil the targets are very low. Unfulfilled targets are the sources of stress for the person. The doer is subject to massive stress in both cases.

Work Abundance

Work abundance is the measure of extra work in the organization to be undertaken by people in the organization. Work abundance is nothing but an extra workload per person. The doer is expected to perform more, with a higher degree of vigour. With the additional work to do, the doer feels the pressure of work and finds it difficult to perform. The result, obviously, is stress. Work abundance implies the following:

1. Additional energy to put into the system
2. Performing at a higher level of output with the same levels of pays, perks and other inputs to the system

The demand for additional energy of the doer is obviously straining to him. Doer feels stressed in the face of the extra work pressure. This coupled with the other factor of performing at no extra benefit would mean that person is under considerable stress. Work abundance thus creates additional stress in the doer. This becomes even more evident when the doer is faced with not only a higher volume of work but also a higher level of quality of the product. It may also be seen as work diversification. Organization may like to offer a framework for diversifying into many other areas of work where the organization does not have any standard measurement of work. Be it increase in absolute workload, increase in the work quality, diversification of work or a combination of these, the doer is in the context of getting into stress. The higher the degree of vulnerability to these, the higher the level of stress is.

REFERENCES

Boone, L. E., and D. L. Kurtz. 1987. *Management*. London: Random House.

French, J.-R. P., and R. D. Caplan. 1973. 'Organisational Stress and Individual Strain'. In *The Failure of Success*, edited by A. J. Marrow. New York: Amacon.

Levinson, H. 1973. 'Problems That Worry Our Executives'. In *The Failure of Success*, edited by A. J. Marrow. New York: Amacon.

Pareek, L. 1981. *ORS Scale, Measuring Role Stress*. Ahmedabad: Indian Institute of Management Ahmedabad.

Porter, L. W., and E. F. Lawler. 1965. 'Properties of Organisation Structure in Relation to Job Attitude and Job Behaviour'. *Psychological Bulletin* 64: 23–51.

Quinn, R. P., S. Seashore, and I. Mangione. 1971. *Survey: Working Conditions*. New York: US Government Printing Office.

CHAPTER 6

WORK-LIFE STRESS
The Human Environment

Human environment is even more important than physical environment. This talks about the likely quality of interpersonal and group interactions in the organization. The broad categories for this are as follows:

TEN FACTORS FOR HUMAN ENVIRONMENT

1. Relationship at work (RW)
2. Scope for career growth (SCG)
3. Adaptability to organizational change (AOC)
4. Authority–responsibility matrix (ARM)
5. Values incongruence (VI)
6. Interpersonal/group communications (IGC)
7. Deficit/abundance of mind energy (DAME)
8. Behaviour restrictions (BR)
9. Degree of autonomy in work (DAW)
10. Flow of learning in organization (FLO)

Out of the 10 factors for human environment, as has been shown above, not all are equally important. The importance of one factor is invariably a function of the locational position, relative to place and timing in organizations. A stressful situation arises on the deviation from the normal or mean position. For each of the 10 factors, the normal or mean position could be understood through an analysis of the individual and the organization. There are situations of conflicts as also congruences for each of the factors. Greater non-congruence leads to larger amounts of stress for the person. The multiplicity of these kinds of situations stresses organizations. A greater number of individuals at stress in the organizations can make the organization more stressed. Otherwise, stressing factors in the system, structures and procedures also create a stressed organization. Now, we shall analyse each of the factors on their merit.

RELATIONSHIP AT WORK

Workplace relationship spans from subordinate to superior relationships through the peers. This can be seen in the following ways:

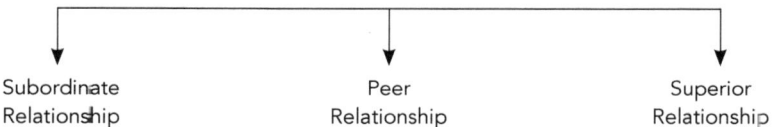

| Subordinate Relationship | Peer Relationship | Superior Relationship |

Subordinate Relationship

Under normal circumstances, the boss is expected to have a good relationship with the subordinates. The subordinate might measure the relationship in terms of the following:

1. Volume of work
2. Frequency of work
3. Value of work
4. Essence of behaviour
5. Human considerations
6. Control–autonomy
7. Learning or career gain

The subordinate relationship is a very important indicator in the workplace. This is supported by views of applied psychology which says that the inherent tendency of a human being is to look upwards always with a view to measure his relative position in any collective or any forum. This is spelled out to express the social position as follows:

Poverty

It is the sense of relative non-possessiveness of resources by people. We do not measure our richness relative to the more underprivileged in society, but rather we measure our poverty by comparison with the richer people in society.

Power/Authority

Power or authority in an organization has got both subjective and objective components. The objective component is the measurable aspect of it, whereas the subjective component is the perception of authority.

At the perceptive level, a subordinate feels like getting more powers, almost equal to the level of the boss. Any shortfall in that may lead to stress.

Subordinates have an inherent tendency to look at
the boss as an equal or less.

If the subordinate fails to have equal or more power in any particular aspect of the work with which he is bestowed, he starts getting depressed in mind, the end product of which is stress. The subordinate, in his subconscious, wants to be treated as the boss by others and as equal by the boss. In social meets and gatherings, the mind of the subordinate will surface. In the work context, the subordinate might hide this drive for a while and behave in a normal manner; yet the subconscious prompts him in the desired manner always. This makes the subordinate depressed.

Control–autonomy is another important concern in the subordinate's life. Whereas the general expectation is greater autonomy and limited control, if it happens, that autonomy decreases constantly but control increases. Higher control and lesser autonomy reduce the degree of motivation to work. A less motivated or less inspired person can hardly contribute to the fullest extent and

Table 6.1 Stressing in Subordinate Relationship

Factors	Normal Expectation	Becomes Stressful When
Volume of work	Moderate or low	High or aggressively high
Frequency of work	Low or very low	High or very low
Value of work	High subjective and moderate objective	Low or very high
Essence of behaviour	Humane	Rough, unfriendly, unscrupulous
Human considerations	Sympathy, friendly, caring, compassionate	Indifferent, arrogant, at enmity
Control–autonomy	Autonomy and greater limited control	Control increases, autonomy decreases
Learning or career gain	Constant learning, undeterred career progression	No learning takes place through work and career progress stops or slows down

cannot enjoy peace at work. Stress continues to pinch in and increases with the persistence of a higher degree of control and lower autonomy. Withdrawal of the control factor or giving autonomy can help remove stress immediately. Persistence is not there for a longer period.

Learning or career gain is considered a very important factor these days. A person's expectation is of a constant scope for learning and undeterred career progression. Learning helps to induce a higher degree of inspiration in the person. A boss who can impart this learning turns into a boss-teacher. Thus, the person is out of the impact of stress. Career gain is another important area of concern. Work that helps attain higher levels in a career is nonstressing. Even if in this case, work volume, frequency, etc., is high, objective work value is also very high and work may not be stressing because of it, leading towards career progression. Learning organizations or learning situations in organizations continuously add factors of stress. This increases stress further when added to career horizons. Prospective career gains ease out the situation through a higher capability of the person. Stress does not go away under the limiting effects of these two factors. It may sometimes happen that the organization is not learning but the boss is; in such an event, the scenario remains the same. A stressed person can cope with stress to a great extent to advance himself and his career.

A person wants a high subjective value and moderate objective value of his work. A lowering of the subjective value of the work or a very high objective value of work creates tension and stress. The creation of stress here is persistent and takes time to return to the normal range of its output when the stressing factors are removed substantially. An inertial phase of stressing remains with work value problems.

The essence of behaviour, as one understands from the terminology, is highly subjective and is remembered by an individual for a longer time. Humane behaviour in organizations has become a scarce thing. Rough, unfriendly and unscrupulous behaviours are most abundant in society and organizations. When we expect humane behaviour but receive inhumane behaviour, we get stressed. Even when the stressors go or are removed, the inertial impact of the spell of stress remains. A transformation of unfriendly, rough, unscrupulous behaviour to humane behaviour may not be able to bring change in the spell of stress. So, a stressed person does not return to the normal state immediately. It takes a lot of time for him to return to normalcy. So, the stress here is for a longer span than the earlier categories

Human considerations are the qualities of interactions revealing the character of the human being. Qualities such as sympathy, friendliness, care and compassion are expected in work life. But quite frequently, these qualities are missing. Indifferent and arrogant attitudes create stress. The return to a friendly, compassionate attitude might prove to be strategic and not acceptable to the people concerned on good faith. People regard these changes sceptically, searching for ulterior motives. Stresses that stand in this category are difficult to remove as once injured, the mind dwells on the injury for a long period. The vibrant memory of the injuries of the mind continues for a longer period, implying a difficult phase for the stressed person. Though the causes no longer persist, stress does not end here. It continues to work in the person and torment him. An arrogant or indifferent person suddenly converting to a friend or sympathetic person creates many doubts, so stress continues to act, to a varying degree, but it does not stop

As shown in Table 6.1, stressing in a subordinate relationship is a function of several factors. The volume of work is one of the most important factors. If the volume is very high or just high, the person immediately feels stressed. He is stressed to the extent of depending upon the volume being high and above his perception. A high volume of work is a load and creates and acts as a burden on the subordinate person. So long as the high volume of work persists, stress will continue, as shown below in Figure 6.1:

As shown in Figures 6.1 and 6.2, high work volume beyond the normal range creates stress. This is smoothly increasing, supernormally, rising more than a proportionate rate with the rising volume of work, and sharply declining to the normal level of stress as soon as work volume returns to the normal level.

The same is the case with the frequency of work. Keeping volume per work constant, if the frequency is changed, we expect

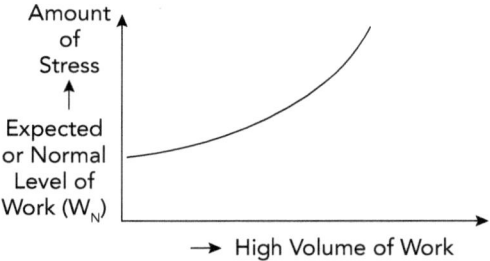

Figure 6.1 Stress–Volume Diagram

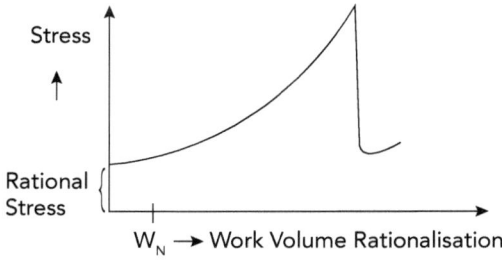

Figure 6.2 Stress–Volume Rationalization Diagram

a change in the measure of stress in the individual. A sharp return of work frequency to the normal level means the stress of a normal measure. The trauma of increasing the output of stress does not remain in the memory beyond a longer period than the normal ones in both the cases of high volume and high frequency of work.

The difference is expected to be experienced with the value of work. Value can be objective as well as subjective.

So far, we have discussed the subordinate relationship at work. Various stressing factors that are present in the subordinate relationship are also present in the peer and superior relationships. Every person is ultimately a subordinate to another person or groups of persons. Thus, the subordinate relationship applies to all. Among the three, besides subordinate relationships, peer relationship creates peer pressure on the person. These are mostly subjective in nature. Peer pressures are the group dynamics in an unrelated or related team where things are mostly remote controlled by the views of the peers. Peer pressures can be stipulated by certain peer qualities such as:

1. Peer jealousy
2. Peer backbiting
3. Conforming to peer identity and peer ego
4. Submitting to peer dynamics

Peer jealousy is very much present in work situations involving personal contacts and interactions. Peer jealousy is a result of peer ego. Lack of an appropriate image, lack of power or position, lack of resources and income and lack of recognition in a broader context create peer jealousy.

SCOPE TO CAREER GROWTH

Many people have observed and experienced that role stress does not always occur and change in the same manner. Stress increases in certain cases and reduces in certain other cases. For example, stress reduces with:

1. Increase in age
2. Increase in the length of service

3. Reduction in the span of control

4. Increase in income

On the other hand, occupational stress increases with hazardous work and with the conflict between work and home demands. Career growth is considered the most important parameter in work life. Expectations develop because of the ultimate prominence given to every aspect of career concerns and concern for relative importance in career accomplishments. Because career is given the utmost importance, any non-fulfilment of career objective leads to stress. Scope for career growth minimizes major parts of work-life stress. Stress reduces with the scope for career growth. Concerns for career growth are expressed through various means and channels. Career growth may be felt in the following ways:

1. speed of growth or growth potential in career

2. quality of growth in career

The concern for career growth sometimes is spelled out in terms of the pace of growth. Someone who is placed in fast-track promotion feels more satisfied than some other who is put on a slow track. The slow track is less attractive than the fast track. In the initial phase or at the level of potential, the fast track is less stressful than the slow track. Actuals differ widely from the features of the potentials; when it comes to the actuals, the demands and pressures of the fast track prove much higher than the demands and pressures of the slow track. Stress is linearly correlated to the demands and pressures of the system which involves the person in work. Obviously, the possibilities of stress in a fast-track growth system are more than the possibilities of stress in a slow track system.

Quality of growth in work life refers to the qualitative changes in the growth. Growth involving wider dispersion in the qualities of the job profile is stressful.

As shown in Matrices 6.1 and 6.2, the pace of career growth and the quality of career growth contribute to various kinds of stress in changing situations.

Q1 shows the case of a high pace of career growth at the potential stage. When at the potential stage, only the blues of career

Low stress (Q1)	Highly stressing but for a short while (Q2)
High stress for a longer period (Q3)	Low stress (Q4)

Growth in work life ↑

Matrix 6.1 The Pace of Career Growth–Stress Analysis

Low stress (G1)	Very low stress, almost stress-free (G2)
High stress (G3)	Moderate stress (G4)

Growth in work life

Career demand   Career overfulfilled
Career expectations

Matrix 6.2 Career Expectation–Quality of Growth Matrix

growth are observed. A person cannot really understand or does not want to understand what sort of work pressures and demands on him would be there during the performance of a high pace job. This helps the person to maintain a satisfactory, even delighting condition. The capability of the person thus increases and greatly reduces the scope for stress

Q2, on the other hand, talks about the actual situation of the high pace of career growth. Being in a high pace of career growth, the person experiences the workload, work pace and demands placed by the elements of work. The pressures and demands placed by a high pace work are highly stressing with the effect being short-lived. A person gets stressed, but immediately afterwards, he regains the power to recover from the trauma considering the potentials of the job. The outcome is expected to be high stress only for a short while.

Q3 discusses the low pace of career growth at potential stages. A low pace of career growth does not delight a person. This immediately causes frustration in the person, a prolonged stay of which causes obvious stress. Q3 combination creates stress for long periods.

Q4 talks about the low pace of work and may create some amount of stress but within a manageable time frame and quantum limit.

As has been seen with the pace of growth, stress also varies with the quality of career growth as shown in Matrix 6.2.

G1 is the case where career expectations are denied but the quality of career growth is high. In this case, the amount of stress generated because of denied expectations is partly offset by the quality of career growth. In practical situations, this might mean the person is denied of due promotion but gets a new job profile that is of higher esteem. Job quality enhancement pleases the person, which greatly offsets the amount of stress generated through the deprivation. The ultimate effect is low stress for the person.

G2 shows the position of high quality in growth as also over-fulfilled expectation. An example of this might be a factory worker getting double promotion in a corporate green chamber. The person having been doubly satisfied forgets about the pressures and burdens of work. Even then some amount of stress pinches him at times. The ultimate result, therefore, stands as very low stress, almost a condition of stress-free.

G3 shows the case of high stress. The condition being the reverse of G2 appears to be more or less the opposite. A person is denied career growth and is put on the low-quality career track. This is one of the most damaging combinations in work life. People become highly frustrated and get into perpetual stress of high magnitude. It is like trauma and becomes difficult for the person to overcome.

G4 signifies another combination of things in work life. Quality of growth being low here, a sense of dissatisfaction remains in the person, biting his mind constantly that generates a significant amount of stress. Whereas overfulfilled expectations act positively to reduce some amount of stress, the ultimate result is a high or moderate level of stress for a longer period.

A study of the organizational character would place the discussion in a proper perspective offering a way out to the basic problems of work-life stress.

ORGANIZATIONAL CHARACTER: AN ENQUIRY INTO THE PHILOSOPHY OF ORGANIZATIONS

The Issue of Organizational Character

Why do organizations exist? The answer may not be homogenous everywhere for each type of organization. One may survive and sustain with the purpose to make one's presence felt by others, another may like to survive to grow in dimension, whereas still others may like to exist to amass material wealth. There could be yet another group that survives and works for others. This group does not want to live for its own sake, but rather, it tries to fulfil a motto whereby it gets joy in the fulfilment of others. 'You grow bigger, you grow beautiful – enjoy by seeing that only' are the words of the hearts of a great many dedicated souls. Organizations grow on their own lines of vision, mission, competence and requirements vis-à-vis the providences of society and the world.

The quest has been primarily sounded by few individuals: 'What am I to do with my life'?, 'why this sort of life'?, 'when shall we reach the summit of fulfilment in life?' Few quests are prominently seen and heard in human contexts. Theorists usually believe that the behaviour of a person reveals the expression of his inner realities. Similarly, the organization is revealed through its behavioural pattern. Behaviour of the organization could be expressed through the set of interactions between an individual and the organization. In these sets of interactions, one could consider the organization as a neuter body or assign personalities to that. A study of the pattern of behaviour by the organization reveals its intrinsic and extrinsic worth and tries to cash in on it with a view to understanding any future course of action or interaction therefrom. A study of the organizational behaviour shows how the behavioural pattern should be designed or followed. In doing so, one loses the human side of the organization by trying to understand its behaviour on a longer term

As in the case of organizations, an individual's behaviour shows the extrinsic, short-term to them. A study of the individual character would obviously show the realms of permanence and long term. It appears at the beginning of an analysis of the philosophy of the organizations that the behaviour of a person or an organization has a longer and transcending dimension—that of character. The basic qualities of individuals come from the character. Character is what gives shape to the attributes of a personality. From character flows the human destiny. An act derives its origin from a thought; a habit from repetitions of the same action. Character is moulded through repeated habits and, finally, habit constitutes the destiny. Why the sense of character becomes important? John Milton hints at the need for character in his magnum opus, *Paradise Lost:*

> *To human Sense the invisible exploits of warring spirits, how without remorse the ruin of so many glorious once and perfect while they stood, how lost* unfold the secrets of another world.

The art and science of character involve discussing the issues of intrinsic factors and external influences in the life of an individual or an organization. An individual is known partly through a few interactions of his/her behaviour but more convincingly through the dynamics of his/her character. A study of the character makes one more revealed to the others. Behavioural inputs certainly corroborate the character of the individual on many occasions and in many incidents, but these do not necessarily unfold the personality. A transparent revelation of the organization shows its strengths or weaknesses. Behaviour, for example, might show certain things which are not the attributes of the personality types or aspects of behaviour that are superimposed or artificially external to the entity; hence, they do not offer the correct picture of the entity. Behaviour that reveals the character is the right one. A study of organizational behaviour, similarly, gives a view about its behaviour. It may be intrinsic or external, but it does not describe the personality fully. A better idea of the entity could be obtained through a study of the organizational character

Organization's Legacy

Chester I. Barnard's great work *The Functions of the Executive* has described the ways and means to develop organizations based on cooperation. Barnard, known as a Closed System Theorist, defines the organization, as mentioned in the discussions on theories of management, as under:

The life of an organisation depends on its ability to secure and maintain the personal contributions of energy necessary to effect its purposes. This ability is a composite of perhaps many efficiencies and inefficiencies in the narrow sense of these words, and it is often the case that inefficiency in some respect can be treated as the cause of total failure, in the sense that corrected success would then be possible. But certainly, in most organisations—social, political, national, religious— nothing but the absolute test of survival is significant objectively, there is no basis for comparison of the efficiencies of separate aspects.

Survival is being seen as the only measure of the efficiency of an organization. The thing is like, 'I win the test of life-therefore I survive'. So, my survival proves my worth.

The question that arises at this point is: 'I survive-it is OK. But what has been the quality of my survival?' In a way, the question hints at the direction of life's journey and the intrinsic qualities in that. The devil and divine both survive during the same period. If survival is the only test, then they don't make any difference in between. On the test of survival, the devil and the divine are treated as the same. But coming to their character, one finds that the devil's utility in the society or the world proves to be unworthy, with likely negative impacts. John Milton's *Paradise Lost* again recounts this point:

For though I fled him angry, yet recalled
To life prolonged and promised race, I now
Gladly behold though but his utmost skirts
Of Glory, and far off his steps adore. (XI–300)

And, by contrast, the character of divine is revealed by Milton as

God is as here, and will be found a sign
Present, and of his presence many a sign
Still following thee, still compassing thee round
with goodness and paternal love, his face
Express, and of his steps the track divine. (XI–350)

Certainly, it makes a difference between the two characters in an organization. The devil character splits, disintegrates, takes one backward and leads to fragments and darkness, whereas the divine character brings in the goodness and paternal love expressed through the face (or the form of the entity) and turns the environment divine. Organizational Ecology discusses certain issues which are better solved through the dominance and interplay of character.

Organizational Ecology

As already mentioned, Chester I. Barnard's views an organisation as a closed type system, with the scope to have meaningful comparisons among different functions of different organizations. Organizations receive support and contributions from their people when their characteristic features find a match and support in the individuals they deal with. The ecology of an organization is tuned by the people inside. Those who work in and with the organization, through their acceptance of it in totality, induce a lot of influence on the systems of the entity. Competition across the boundaries of the organization does take place in the case of it being able to develop congruence between the set of attributes it possesses and the continuous impact with the interactions from various quarters - the individuals, the collectives, etc. Ecology is the climate that the organization has been endowed with, carrying it constantly, with a view to foster its way ahead. Again, referring to Chester I. Barnard, about the commercial and non-commercial types of organizations, we note the following.

> It is said that a commercial organisation cannot survive unless its income exceeds its outgoings, a statement that begs the point. It is only true if no one will contribute the deficit in commercial goods for non-commercial reasons. But this infrequently occurs. Finally pride, philanthropic motives, etc. often induce economic contributions for non-commercial motives that enable an organisation that is economic in character to survive. And the fact is plain that organisations in large numbers that are unsuccessful economically nevertheless continue to exit, whatever the motives.

Organizations that bulge in the population do get the effect of ecologies. G. R. Carroll, an organizational ecologist of repute, argues as under:

The characteristic growth of trajectory (railroads etc.) reflects the operation of opposing processes in legitimation and completion. At low density, growth in numbers mainly legitimates a population and the organisational form it uses. But when density is high in relation to resources, increase in density mainly strengthens the process of completion.

The density as we are talking about could be of individuals grouped across certain attributes that they possess. It could be on the broad categories also. Structural similarity prior to analysing the density of attributes would be vital. It is like the urge to find members who could be branded as nobles possessing good qualities.

They could be seen as honest, hardworking, committed, cooperative, selfless, compassionate, diligent, sincere, positive and goal-oriented. Each one of these values or any mix of these could be taken as units, and a cluster of people around which each unit could be assessed. It is based on the clusters of values that one can form a structure. A structure based on a cluster value like that would give an ideal combination, and this is recounted as a dominant value. An organization is encountered with this dominant value to form new value through the synthesis between the existing ones and the new ones. Dominant values highlighted in this cluster-value analysis show the type of the unit and then pick up on the right mix of its formation. Ultimate structures of the organizations are based on these types and structures. At this point, an analysis between an organization behaviour in a particular characteristic way and the industry behaving in another way proves important.

A study of the structural eco-dynamics of organizations by Caves and Porter (1977, 92–93) argues that

> Because of their structural similarity, (industry) group members are likely to respond in the same way to disturbances from inside or outside the group, recognizing their independence closely and anticipating their reactions to one another's moves quite accurately. Profit rates may differ systematically among the groups making up an industry, the differences stemming from competitive advantages that a group may posses against others. The industry's profits and (perforce)

the average level of its group's profit depends on the general structural traits of the industry and also the internal heterogeneities that identify the groups.

This aspect of group-member interaction has its legacy to individuals also. Within the organization, this is accomplished partially through the dynamics of power that they are into. Discussion on the real nature of power within organization continue until an agreed scientific decision is arrived. This could be expressed in specific terms as:

> Power is exercised when A participates in the making of decisions that have an impact. But power is also exercised when A devotes his energies to creating or reinforcing social and political values and institutional practices that limit the scope of the political process to public consideration. Of only those issues which are comparatively innocuous to A, To the extent that A succeeds in doing this, B is prevented, for all practical purposes, from bringing to the fore any issues that might in their resolution be seriously detrimental to A' s set of preferences.

Exercise of power is the function of the set of attributes the individual possesses vis-à-vis that of the organization. As we have already mentioned about some of the personal attributes, there is a need to identify an appropriate set of organizational attributes that fit into the design of the system. A system is a composite of attributes that figures in the organization through synchronization of the personal attributes and organizational attributes. Daniels and Daniels (1993) in their pioneering work on Global Vision have identified 10 attributes that make up a global vision as well as go a long way to creating the mindset that each individual working in a global corporation must have. There has been a clear shift in the focus: from the modem perspective to a supra-modem perspective. The issues highlighted by Daniels and Daniels are as follows:

1. From a geographic to a business concept
2. From a focus on centralization versus decentralization to a business 'any place'

3. From a mechanistic to a holistic view of business
4. From isolationism to low or non-existent boundaries
5. From not invented 'here' to network of trust
6. From mere physical geographic presence to acceptance by the local culture
7. From centralized controllers to core management
8. From duplication of resources to taking advantage of economies of scale
9. From vertical 'stovepipe' communications to communication networks
10. From a short-term view to a long-term view

The analysis of the above-quoted attributes put forward by Daniels underlines a general trend in the expectations towards the corporate mindsets or attributes the process could be considered as the identification of the attributes in the individual personalities and then seeing them to cascade down to the ground realities of the organization. A transition from geographic to the business concept, centralization to decentralization and mechanistic to holistic approaches requires a personality type and a character that proves a long-term effect for the organization. Again, referring to other attributes like creating boundaryless organization, a network of trust, acceptability, establishing core management, mass production, communications network and a long-term focus require a set of values that individuals can have as characteristic features. Globalization means extending the reach and presence. Universalizing the corporation would demand a universal mind and the characteristic type of individual for universal corporations. Creating and catering for homogeneous products and services demand a sustainable character of the organization. Certain questions that are relevant here could be listed as follows:

Questions	Answers
1. Whose organization is this?	Human's
2. Who are the beneficiaries?	The global person
3. What is the guiding rule of the business?	Trust

4. What is the essential type and framework of the organization?	Universal
5. What is the guiding philosophy of the entity?	Observation: An organization with integrated personalities, remembering that it can prove to be worthy of perpetually answering the questions above.

In Search of Bliss

Why is there the need for the study of character?

The response obviously comes from the basic urge or tendency in the human system. Why do I live life; why shall the organized entity survive and grow? The answer would be Bliss, Bliss & Bliss. Man survives to have a taste of or reaching the realm of bliss. In the words of Pascal (Pascal, 169) 'Man wishes to be happy and only exists to be happy and cannot wish not to be happy'.

According to Kant, 'he (man) never can say definitely and consistently what it is that he really wishes. He cannot determine with certainty what would make him truly happy; because to do so he would need to be omniscient'.

Starting from the principles of Pascal and then coming to the point highlighted by Immanuel Kant, we find in the quest for human happiness comes first as the thing to each but then systematic probing into this leads to the logical culmination of the same-where a transcendence to the ultimate truth or omniscient becomes a prelude to that. The active principle of this is highlighted by Socrates in Plato's *Phaedrus,* saying, 'I must first know myself ... to be curious about that which is not my concern, while I am still in ignorance of my own self would be ridiculous'.

It is that identifying the realms of the inner worlds of human beings, an appeal to the understanding or realization of the truth within, proves worth to fulfil the quest of a human being. In the words of Ananda K. Coomaraswamy, 'If it is to nourish and make the best part of us grow, as plants are nourished and grow in suitable soils, it is to the understanding and not to fine feelings that an appeal must be made.'

It appears from this discussion that in our quest for Bliss, we get happiness and are immersed in it. Happiness, in the usual sense of the term, gets material fulfilment for the persons but leaves open the inner realms. At this point, quoting E. F. Schumacher would be appropriate. Schumacher (1977, 147) in his famous work *A Guide for the Perplexed* mentions:

> Everything in this world around us must be matched, as it were, to enhance our level of Being we have to adopt a life-style conducive to much enhancement, which means one that grants us lower nature just the attention and care it requires and leaves us with plenty of time and free attention for the pursuit of our higher development.

Blissful Character

Schumacher rightly points out that enhancing the level of Being demands a conducive lifestyle. This presupposes granting of just attention to lower forms of demand and then devoting adequate time to the development of the higher qualities. A blissful character is stress-free.

ADAPTABILITY TO ORGANIZATIONAL CHANGE

There could be many factors of changes. An adaptive person can be expected to be positive towards the direction of changes. However, the conditions of adaptability are dependent functions of the quality and face of change. Individuals become suspicious of the process of change when the process of change becomes abrupt and cursive to the individual. Making people adaptive to change is very important for any corporation. Resistance to change creates problems for the individual as well as the organization. The analysis of adaptability may be made based on certain accepted models of the process of change. The Force-Field Theory of Kurt Lewin could be the basis of the model of change process. Lewin identifies driving forces as the positives and the restraining forces as the negatives. According to Lewin, a person's behaviour in the organization or a group context is the result of a dynamic equilibrium between the driving and the restraining forces. There are push-pull effects of the driving and the restraining forces. Lewin identifies multiple causes of the driving as well as the restraining forces. He differentiates forces for change from forces for maintaining the status quo. According to him, forces for change are as follows:

1. New technology
2. Better raw materials
3. Competition from other groups
4. Supervisor pressures

Forces maintaining the status quo, Lewis mentions the need of the following:

1. Group performance norms
2. Fear of changes
3. Member complacency
4. Well-learned skills

The impact of the push and pull of the driving and the restraining forces are the changes in the system. This process of change incorporates a shift in the level of performance. Changes are normally aimed at a higher level of performance for the person in the organization. The processes of change as advised by many authors for both the planned as well as unplanned changes are as follows:

1. Approaches to structural change
2. Organizational change
3. Changes in technostructure
4. Changes in people

For an effective process of change, the common steps that are involved are as follows:

Unfreezing

Changing

Refreezing

Unfreezing: is a step where the need for the change mode is felt by people.

Changing: is the phase spearheaded by the change agents. Change agents are the leaders of change. They change the attitudes, values, beliefs, approaches, cultures of the organization with respect to those of the persons' and previous levels of accomplishments. These changes in attitude, values and beliefs foster effective transformation through identification with those and Internalization of those changes thus internalized. Make sure to effectively implement the things in a system for perpetual fulfilment of the organizational goals both in the short run as well as in the long run.

Refreezing: is the reinforcement of the new behavioural pattern into the norms and practices through replacement of the old ones through replacement and support mechanisms.

Lewin made thorough studies to present the cases of change as also to offer models of change He found the efforts of changes failing because of two reasons

1. Attitudes of the persons in the chain of change
2. Behaviour of the person resulting from the interaction to initiate change

Studies by Edgar H. Schein and others offer an extension of Lewin's Field–Force Theory and exposition. Schein believed in the process of unfreezing then changing then again refreezing as the terms have) been defined earlier.

The problems that arise with these approaches to define the process of change in terms of the parameters lay down above lie with capability. It may be said that capability is difficult to understand. In view of this problem, there is a need to understand the process of change in the manner in which should be.

Process of Change and Its Management

Changes take place in two distinctly different aspects of management functions and processes. Changes are basically due to two factors:

1. Extrinsic factors of change
2. Intrinsic factors to change

The capability of the pressures of change and its management depend upon the individual factors of those involved in the process of transformations.

Lewin's model as discussed earlier fails to identify intrinsic or extrinsic factors to the person. Whereas the factors relating to structural changes, organizational change, changes in technostructure and changes in people refer to the extrinsic factors. The intrinsic factors are specific to different people. All changes fostered from outside do seek support, recognition and concurrence from the inner self of persons involved in the process. Adaptability can be achieved through the concurrence of the inner to the outer stimuli. On full accomplishment, the person occupies a position at 'A' as shown in Figure 6 3. A person has the scope to develop capability through strategies or efficiently managing himself. The position 'B' as shown in Figure 6.3 describes the plight of a person faced with negative effects of the external stimuli. In this analysis, we assume that the external stimuli index to change is linearly related to stress. This means that all aspects of the linear indicators to change are stressing. They create stress irrespective of the directions of change. Negative external stimulus, then, means a set of changes that might be less stressing in the gamut of the works that are undertaken. Adaptability to change as shown in Figure 6.3 is the result of the factors intrinsic to the person. Adaptability is near zero for a

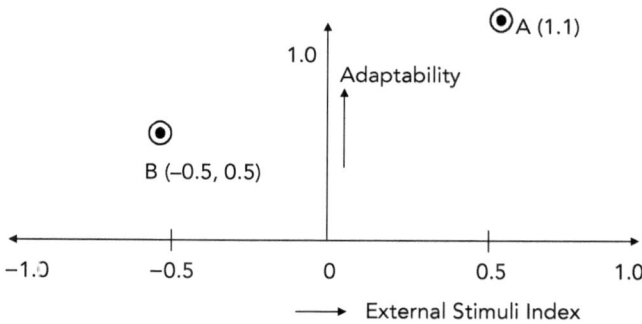

Figure 6.3 Adaptability–External Stimuli Index Matrix

person who is broken by stress or less in the strength of personality to cope; the higher the strength of personality, the higher is the adaptability to change. Personality types may be explained to prove the same. In *Mother Leadership*, Banerjee (1998) has developed the concept of *sthitaprajna* manager. *Sthitaprajna* means a equipoised personality. A person who develops a state of equanimity in all situations is above the influences of the stressors.

An analysis of the adaptability based on the traits of personality does require appropriate scaling of personality starting from one end of it to the other. Figure 6.4 shows the relationship between adaptability and the index of individuality. Individuality is shown extending from fragmented being who is fully exteriorized to the *sthitaprajna* who is equipoised in all situations. A fragmented personality is akin to the external influences and is swayed by the external incidents, with a potential to affect him.

Adaptation becomes a far-flung thing to him because of the inherent propensities to crave for things one after the other. Seeking leads to frustrations and ultimately stress.

A fragmented being is always under the spell of desire and want. He is a perpetual seeker. As he seeks things one after the other, chances are high that he is denied the fulfilment of the

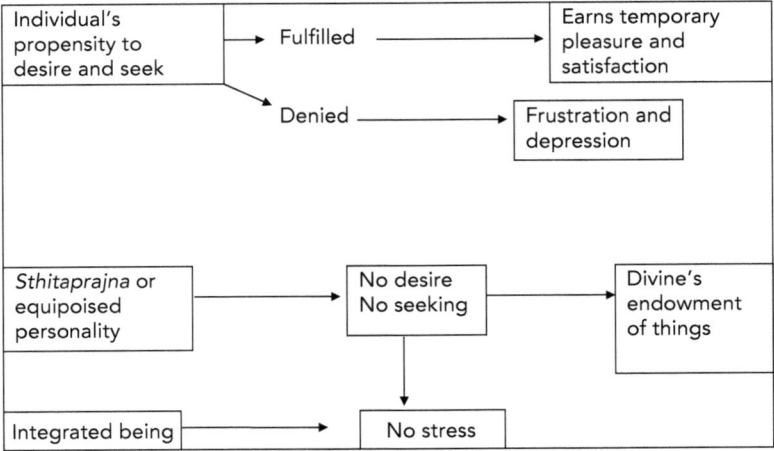

Figure 6.4 Stress in the Different States of the Personality

STRESS MANAGEMENT THROUGH MIND ENGINEERING

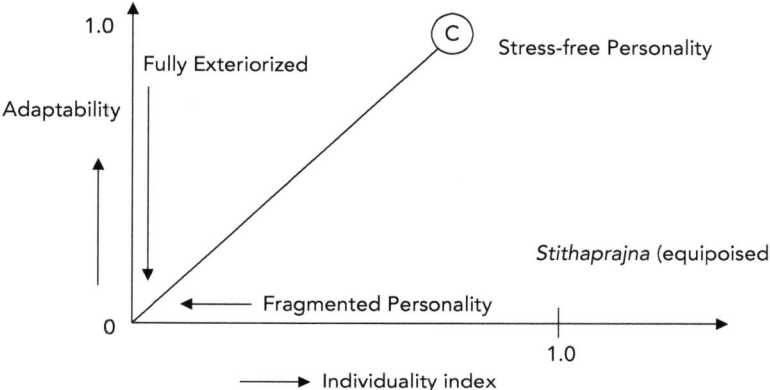

Figure 6.5 Adaptability–Individuality Index

desires. One desire fulfilled means the birth of another leading to the rise of further chances to be denied fulfilment. Individuals thus denied the fulfilment of desires get frustrated and depressed. This depression and frustration ultimately lead to stress. An integrated being, on the other hand, is beyond this kind of frustration. As desires and seeking are absent, individuals can get into a condition of indifference to all possible situations. He does not seek anything. So, the question of him getting the desire fulfilled does not arise. He is all the same in all situations, that is, he is equipoised.

Seek Not Avoid Not

A *sthitaprajna* has realized the real essence of life. He does not seek anything, but at the same time, he does not avoid anything also. He is not a grabber of opportunities, but the fair opportunities reaching his ends are cordially welcomed and accepted with gratitude. He does not show the strength of his ego through the harsh denial of things. Seek not; avoid not remains the mantra of his life. A *sthitaprajna* believes in the following:

1. Truthful thoughts, perceptions and actions.
2. Fairness in all sorts of deals and interactions.
3. Openness to the maximum extent (transparency).

4. Full of respect and gratitude.
5. Full of compassion.
6. Friendliness to all, no enmity. Even if he is to fight, wage a war, he does it as a destined duty without having any malice to the opponent.
7. Forgiveness to the wretched.
8. Honesty in his behaviour.
9. Dignity of life in all situations.
10. Cooperation but not compromise.
11. Does not believe in the predominance of the self ego. Rather he sees the divine's hand in all works or deeds. So, his ego is gradually diluted.
12. Above selfishness always.
13. He believes himself as nothing but an embodiment of the divine. He operates on the broadness of the divine and is in a position to embrace all.

AUTHORITY–RESPONSIBILITY MATRIX

All theories of organization discuss the problems of authority and responsibility. Whereas authorities vary with different factors of the organizations, responsibility may also vary due to those factors or different combinations of them. The objective of every organization is to achieve an obvious harmony between authority and responsibility. But one of the most important problems that organizations are faced with is a mismatch between authority and responsibility. Situations of authority keeping parity or showing dissonance with responsibility are worth discussing to understand the spell of stress if it is there. The situations, as mentioned, can be captioned as below:

1. $A = R$ (balanced monolithic management)
2. $A > R$ (authority-centred management)
3. $A < R$ (responsibility-centred management)

where 'A' stands for some measures of authority and 'R' stands for the set of responsibilities that the person is endowed with

According to the prevailing views of the management, authorities could be categorized among the followings:

Line authority

Staff authority

Functional authority

While examining the conditions of match or mismatch between authority and responsibility, the question of the types of authority remains important. Line authority demands a set of responsibilities that suits or fits into the line functions. Similar is the case with two others. But problems arise when expectations vary. The higher the divergence, the greater is the scope for such problems.

Balanced Monolithic Management (A = R)

This occurs when the extent and quality of authority match with the extent and quality of responsibility. This being an ideal situation is hardly seen in organizations except for the few well-knit ones. Deviations from this either creates:

1. An authority-centred enterprise
2. A responsibility-centred enterprise

Authority-centred enterprises have a bias in the authority. Much of authority and less of responsibility make this type. The other type is the responsibility-centred enterprise, where too many responsibilities create imbalance without having matching authority. Both these situations are prone to cause stress.

Authority-centred Management (A > R)

As has been mentioned earlier, line, staff and functional authorities create differential positions.

Line authority is enjoyed by the managers to maintain the chain of command for achieving the organizational goals. Staff authority is supportive and advisory to the line authority advising on the protection of organizational goals through the effective expression of the chain of commands.

Functional authority represents the authority of the staff members of one department on those of other departments to finally fulfil the corporate objective and organizational goal.

It can be seen from the foregoing explanations that line authority expects a set of responsibilities that allows and helps the manager fulfil the company objective through observance of the unity of commands. Authority-centred organization lacks in the rigour of responsibility for line people. Line authority is higher than responsibility. Much of the authority is not reflected through matching responsibilities the scope for the degeneration of discipline and order in the organization. There are abundant examples of public sector organizations in India. Line executives seldom have adequate responsibilities to prove the effectiveness of that. This factor helps degenerate the order into chaos and confusion, leading to a stressful condition for the people working in the organization.

Similar is the case with a staff function. Staff functions naturally are contented with related and matching responsibilities. A person discharging staff functions can seldom accept line responsibilities in good spirit. For a staff function, line responsibility is surely a burden and is disturbing to the person. This situation has got two different derivatives:

1. It motivates the person
2. It stresses the person

Staff function with responsibility motivates the person until a certain level beyond which it appears as a stressor.

Figure 6.6 clarifies the relationship. At the FC level of staff functions, the stress curve shows a level of responsibility equal to RC. At this level of responsibility, the person has no grievance whatsoever. Indifference to stress is the key feature of this point, SC. Above SC, we get into the zone of stress, whereas below SC, the zone bounded by the points RC and FC show a different feature. Within this zone, the responsibilities are more glorious than the functional requirements. This goes a long way to motivate people. With responsibilities overshadowing the functional requirement, people feel elated and motivated.

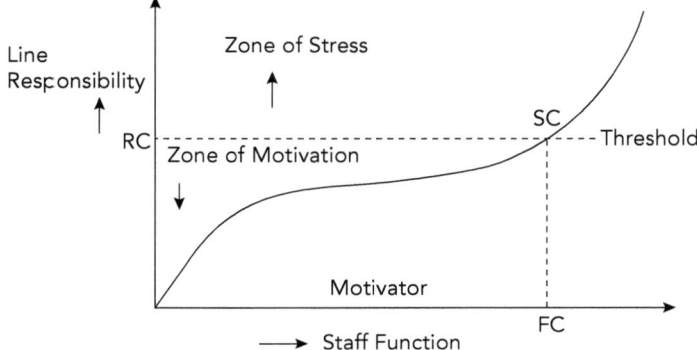

Figure 6.6 Stress/Motivation from: Functions and Responsibilities

VALUES CONGRUENCE

For a stress-free environment, values congruence is essential for organizations. Incongruence in values brings in industrial conflict and a lack of homogeneous relationships. In most cases, industrial conflict arises because of two factors:

1. The objective condition and terms/expectations of the job
2. Values incongruence between the person and the rest of the group

In this section, we shall discuss the causes of industrial conflicts and their impacts and remedies by offering a new idea about the problems of values incongruence leading to a stressful situation.

Conflicts arise not only in the activities but also in the thoughts and their applications. There is no common reason for any conflict in industrial enterprises. It is the attitude to the work or the work itself that proves to be important. Conflicts prevail between the manager and the managed, worker and the supervisor, subordinate and the superior; one department or division and the other, one company and the other, one industry or one regime and the other and one identity and the other. Conflicts arising out of values incongruence lead to conditions of stress, turbulence and sometimes chaos. This may affect growth or lead to decay or at least some change in the design and pattern of few organizations. Conflict causes destruction in some situations, whereas in some other cases, it contributes to the identification and pursuit of a new stream of activities. In many cases, conflict arises because of the emphasis or love of one's own choices preferences, points of view and one's emotions over others. Any two objects or personalities meeting each other may like to do that in a few ways or fashions:

1. Friendly interaction = cooperation
2. Incongruent interaction = conflict

Conflicts may or may not always lead to stress. Certain varieties, degrees, combinations and levels of frequency lead to stress. Stress is the result of sustained conflict, in most of cases, and some of the elements of conflict in many cases when they are intrinsically repeated. Interactions normally turn into conflict in the absence of a proper understanding of the points of view of the other side. Norms of cooperation or the spirit of discord and imbalance create stress. This could be triggered by either the person or the organization or both simultaneously.

Interactions being the driving force, the situation is explained on the basis of the degree of understanding the other side of the spectrum where interactions do take place. When understanding the other side as well as when the degree of interactions is poor, we come across a potential conflict. With the rise of the degree of interactions, the incipient conflict turns into an actual conflict.

	Poor Interactions	High
High Understanding	Good wishes, Inbuilt cooperation (inspired executor, trusted operator)	Full and active cooperation (scopes to motivation)
Poor	Probable conflict (thinly spread stress)	All-out conflict (immediate stress)

Figure 6.7 Interactions–Understanding Matrix

Source: 'Divine Values for Conflict-free Enterprises', a paper by the author at an International Symposium on 'Managing Conflict' held in India during 1999.

High interactions coupled with poor levels of understanding of the other side lead to the situation of an all-out conflict. This makes the situation topsy-turvy. In this situation, there is only conflict and less cooperation. With the increase in understanding of the other side, at the level of poor interaction, it is the good wishes or the potential cooperation that are perceived only. At this level of high understanding of the other side, with the rise in the degree and levels of interactions, gradually we get full and active cooperation. Whereas conflict breeds stress, cooperation tames it.

Now that it is felt, in most of the occasions, conflict is the lack of understanding the other side involved in the interaction—a question may be raised at this point as to why this lack of understanding. This discussion presupposes the implications of conflict being significant to the enterprises. There may be few answers to the question, 'Why not understand the other side'? as follows:

1. Highly egoistic
2. High self-interest
3. High desire and other negative emotions of life
4. Myopic vision of the world of interactions
5. Blind affiliation to one
6. Lack of knowledge of the other (lack of knowledge)
7. Fragmentalism

There could be many more situations or occasions of getting into conflicts. One is prone to conflicts when one finds that through conflicts, he or she is going to get some mileage in certain areas or aspects of his or her existence. Conflict might help in any way to satisfy any aspect of the being to the extent possible and feasible. Through conflicts, one gets those things she or he longed for. As mentioned already, the situations of conflict might have been nourishment to the ego of the person. A highly egoistic person might get a feeling that only through an effective conflict, and the consequential gains in that would satisfy her or his guiding ego. The likely mindsets are: 'I am Mr. so and so—who the hell you are to conflict with me?' I will either finish you or be perished'. In this situation of conflict, either side suffers from the strains of the final rounds. Examples are around trade union-management conflicts particularly in the sunset industries haunted by aggressive trade union movements. Conflicts of this type lead to an either/or situation or exist/perish situation and cannot be considered as good. This breeds stress for both the unionized people as well as the management.

The Self-blinds

Selfish drives always lead to conflicts. Conflicts in the marketplace are of this type. The market is infested with multiple units of high self-interests, each trying to occupy the grounds of the other—leading to a war of interests. Conflicting interests in the market take all possible measures to win the battles. Offensive approaches to the market and marketing are valued as the most effective approach to enterprises. It appears to the enterprises that short-term gains would necessitate them to undertake the course of conflict both at the external and internal aspects of enterprising. This attitude to corporate interactions has arisen as a result of the continuous suggestions made by the behavioural scientists and marketing counsels. The behavioural scientists think that up to a certain stage of its setting in, conflict results in terms of enhancing productivity or efficiency in the corporation. Figure 6.8 shows the relationship between conflict and productivity in corporate organizations. This shows that initially, in the absence of conflict, productivity is very low. As and when conflict increases, productivity also increases. Phase I talks about getting results through a measured degree

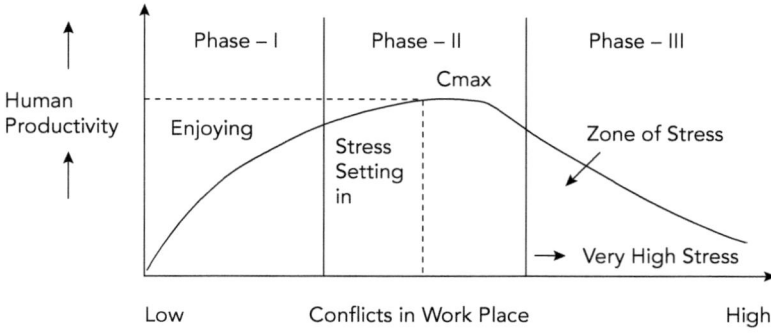

Figure 6.8 Conflict Productivity for Study of Stress

of conflict. Faith in this kind of behaviour talks about the belief that people do not want to give production on their own. A limited degree of conflict goes a long way to make them productive. Phase II shows the maturity level of productivity triggered by conflict up to the point Cmax, productivity increases at different paces, but beyond this point, it reduces substantially. The sharp decrease in productivity is more rigorously caught in Phase III. Here we find aggressive conflict leads to the crumbling down of productivity

The view of the reliance of behavioural scientists (Figure 6.8) on the role of conflict is that they ignore the impact of conflict at different levels. In order to comprehend this dimension, let us try to understand its scope and impact. A real-life case would help us have a feel of the pinch of conflict also.

CASES: THE MONKEY MANAGER

MK, herself a social scientist, was appointed as a lecturer in applied sociology at M3, a business school of repute, by her former teacher's colleague CN, the director of M3. CN, an ardent supporter of and believer in the concepts and practices of social and behavioural science, used to deliberately infuse conflict between the management and the faculty and also among the faculty. He was of the impression that the dynamics as shown in Figure 6.8 would apply to his business school very well, particularly with respect to the members of the faculty.

CN, a dynamic person, was highly egoistic and would expect personal esteem and recognition for every act of him or his team. He had a mix of good and bad behaviours of high degree, unpredictably present now and then. The management of M3 had only some amount of working faith in CN. The belief of CN in the scope and potentials of conflict in delivering productivity made him an autocrat in the guise of a democrat. A very high degree of vigilance and monitoring of the activities of the faculty led to the ruining of the faculty morale in general and weak minds in particular. Mutual trust was lost in the organization.

MK was vehemently attacked by CN in one of his faculty meetings. CN had caused MK not to be able to deliver goods on the 'Social Development of the MBA students'. Though it is a known fact in the organization that every step of action initiated by the faculty is not only approved and endorsed by CN, he influenced all the decisions. The faculty's intellectual liberty is also a myth, forget about the operational liberty, for them. CN did not understand that the drawback lay in the behavioural postulates and approaches to the war on social development in the course of action undertaken by MK. Besides, nothing was measured either to show whether social-behaviour of an average MBA student had improved or not. MK was made responsible for this and was profusely scolded by CN; the result of these kinds of situations was a psychological breakdown for MK. MK being a lady with a sensitive mind could not withstand the bum of the fire in CN's words pouncing on her and she resigned. It was on the verge of the vacation for summer that MK was asked to resign. People in the company realized the game. The juniors felt this as the management's game to force people to fly away before the long holidays. They are short-term oriented and want to get people on shorter terms- thinking that the vacation period should not be given to the faculty as they don't deliver tangible outputs during that period for the institute. CN believes in the opposite of it. When the junior members of the faculty were scared, the seniors felt disillusioned finding it difficult to push the way of the institute through. The institute reached a crossroad of either getting crushed or having a revamp. MK, however, got her chance elsewhere. Later, CN was removed. The person who had replaced CN followed the advice of a senior professor to take back MK at the middle level.

The case of MK-CN ends up with many speculations and multiple possibilities. The theory of measured conflict for corporate results pushes everyone to disillusionment. The ultimate effect is high levels of stress for the person who is a party to the conflict and moderate or low levels of stress for others.

Figure 6.9 shows the situations of the individual goal with some divergence from the company goals. The figure shows three different situations or cases. In case I, the individual has an inclination of Q1 with the company goal. The personality type is such that it can be made to yield results with increased doses of stress or conflict. The second type talks about types of personalities who are prepared to endure and tolerate stress and conflict until the

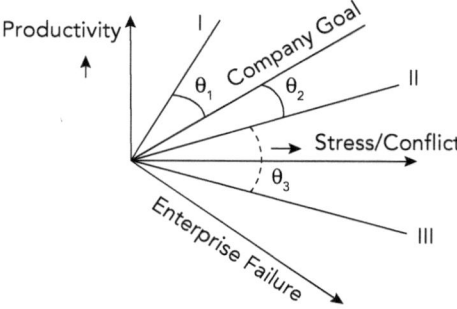

Figure 6.9 Conflict–Productivity through Goal Congruence

end of it. In this case, since the company applied stress or conflict in a measured dose, the degree and magnitude of stress shall lie in phase II of Figure 6.8 as shown earlier. The third type is an inclination of Q3, which indicates that the company goal breaks with the company. The personality types have been explained more elaborately in the matrix as shown in Figure 6.10. Productivity triggered by calculated conflict in the scales of tolerance has been shown here. Three types of personalities P_1, P_2 and P_3 have distinct features different from each other. The first type P_1 could be depicted as Trs with dominant T-attributes. The second one P_2 is dominant R-type, and the third one P_3 is dominant S-type. P_1 has a low tolerance and is a quick changer by responding to the external stimuli at their onset. R-type shows an aggressive attitude

High			Low
P_1 T-type	P_2 R-type	P_3 S-type	
P_{RS} High Stress	Rushers	S_{RT} No Stress	Conflict
Quick Adopters Stress	R_{ST} Restlessness	Waiters Stress	High
Low			
Low	Tolerance	High	

Figure 6.10 Productivity–Conflict Personality Conjoint Analysis for Stress

and ignores the increased levels of stress or conflict. In this case, increased degrees of stress or conflict fail to evoke a productive response from the individuals. The third type SRT represents an extreme variety that is indifferent to the outside stimuli. This type breaks with the parent or the company as soon as there is a sharp change in the levels of stress or conflicts. TRS and SRT are high stressors RST represents a restless condition, stress levels for quick adopters and waiters are low.

This analysis tends to prove that conflict creates the most stress. RST and SRT are the real contributors to productivity in organizations. It is seen that through conflict, an organization loses its cream and focus; hence, there is the need for conflict-free organizations.

The Indian Way to Handle Conflict

We have described so far the behavioural ways to handle conflict. The basic assumption that conflict, in its measured dose, is productive holds good only for laggards and poor performers. A felt and real deficit is, in most of the cases, made good by people through personalised interaction, aiming at satisfying men of power. This is why conflict or stress in measured doses yields good results. The rule applies to those lying at the end of the productive spectrum. For them, productivity enhancement means a lot but only insignificant things or insignificant changes to the organizations.

Conflict can be better handled from a different perspective if personalities are explained from their three different types. The personality types have dominant attributes as shown in Table 6.2.

Table 6.2 Attributes of S-R-T Types of Personalities

S-Type (SRT)	R-Type (RST)	T-Type (TRS)
Continence	Dynamism	Indolence
Forbearance	Anger	Gluttony
Truthfulness	Envy	Sloth
Patience	Jealousy	Idleness

(Table 6.2 Contd.)

(Table 6.2 Contd.)

S-Type (SRT)	R-Type (RST)	T-Type (TRS)
Tolerance	Backbiting	Procrastination
Honesty	Conflicting	Lust
Sincerity	Covetousness	Vacillating
Cooperation	Crookedness	Greedy
Cleanliness	Stealing	Selfishness
Sacrifice	Lying	Slave mind

Table 6.3 S-R-T Matrix for Stress Analysis

S	R	T
High productivity, sustainability, long-term results (system crumbles to form a new one)	Moderate productivity through turbulence; Enduring employee	Productivity under strain only; Timid employee in a caring organization
High market share, but moderate concern for people Moderate concern for production	Short termism; tolerant person in a tolerant system; Dynamism; moderate flexibility	Chaos and turbulence, high risk associated with low productivity Productivity through volatility.
Death of potentiality; system not congenial to growth; Productivity through change/ employee replacement	Rigid command and control; Inactive participation; Conflict-fostered organization	Inertial movement; all-out conflict from the employee as also the organization.
S	R	T

Attributes falling under each category could be considered as the dominant representative of the type and a combination of one with the others are represented as shown in the S-R-T matrix analysis.

Company Types

The above matrix shows various types of combinations between and among the individual and the organization. An S-type of organization meets an S-type of employee together to gain S-type of outputs. An R-type of organization gives outputs of R-type. Similarly, a T-type of person gives T-type of outputs through interactions with a T-type of organization.

These three types of personalities have been shown as types I, II and II in Figure 6.10. Combinations other than (SS), (RR) and (TT) do lie in the vicinity of the line but within the plane of references; it emerges from this discussion that conflict has a very limited scope to yield results. Rather, it is prone to stress to the detriment of the person as well as the organization

Transition of Stressful to Stressless Condition through Culture of Values

It has been observed that human values are basically *rajas*-driven. These values are controlled by the self-initiatives in the realm of selfish interests. They are always propelled by selfish interest and driven by dynamic aspects of it, like greed, anger, envy, gluttony and covetousness. Corporate enterprises accept, in most cases, these as the dominant values, and it is because of these that an individual establishes his or her worth, at times, at the cost of others. Aggressive self-interest of one creates a condition and situation of conflict when it meets that of another; one's objective being to satisfy his selfish drive and fulfil that in the light of his/her own chosen ways, the same can be a vociferous enemy to the other. Conflict is inevitable when we give value to the *rajas* and *tamas* qualities.

As mentioned earlier, dominant quality types emerge through the combinations of S, R, T and Srt, Rst, Tsr—this shows our corporations are mostly Rst or *rajas*-driven and look for the results through the *rajas*-qualities.

A transition from *rajas*-driven to the *sattwa*-driven quality makes the organization reach a situation of getting results from self-motivators. People of this type ignore the external conditionalities and work on their own, conflict in a measured dose fails to prove its position here because they have developed the capacity to absorb stress and endure conflict. *Sattwa* dominated people embody the divine qualities in them and turn the organization into one dominated by divine qualities also. Gradually, as more and more people do adopt divine values, the organization slowly adopts and initiates a sharp change in its outlook and creates a new ambiance to grow. If we refer to Figure 6.9, we find that the individual dynamics shall follow the third axis, and productivity and growth shall take place through the self-initiative of the people with divine qualities.

Indian organizations need to review their position in this context to see the small impact that conflict has instead on productivity and growth—it takes away the productivity. A conflict-free organization offers the ideal environment to grow through the positive participation of people with divine values.

INTERPERSONAL GROUP COMMUNICATIONS

Communication has been spelt out as an understanding between and among the people partaking in the interactions. Certain types of communications are there which derives from the compulsive impulse. Certain other varieties are there which could be termed as spontaneous communications. A star communicator is taken as a leader, at least, apparently. But problems arise in the long term if contents are really missing or lacking; those who have good communication quite often outdo others with much superior knowledge but low communication skill. Communication could be treated as an instrument to interact, sustain and win. That is why it is frequently used as a tool to achieve certain ends in a group or individual context. With competitions growing at a rapid pace, communication is becoming increasingly important.

Communication has been seen by many as the tool to share with or impart to another one's thoughts and information in order to obtain the desired response. Its scope is not only to share thoughts and information but also to sell ideas. In modern organizations of sales and marketing, communication proves to be even more important. The existence, growth and sustenance of organizations depend upon the modes and contents of the communication. It is hardly possible for a modern leader to turn a person into a follower unless efficient communication has taken place. Problems arise in the matching of the mode and contents of communications with the conditions that prevail in the place where the communication process has been initiated. The concept of total communication has become popular. This means using all possible means to communicate the message without any kind of gap or lags in between. Total communication is also seen as total integration and coherence between and among various services. If it is seen that the message conveyed is one and the facts are different, then the very purpose of communication is lost. This situation goes against the very purpose and essence of communication. A small case will explain this point more clearly.

The Case of Cyberage Manager

The Institute of Management Programmes (IMP) was running a master's programme in management. The third batch was out in the job market. The institute has passed through phases of ups and downs with the board of academic directors having been reconstituted very frequently. The student's enrolment in the institute fell short of the strength sanctioned by the government. The first batch had only one-fifth of the sanctioned strength, the second batch one-half and the third and fourth batches also around the same strength. While the admission process for the fourth batch was in process, the lukewarm response made the institute rethink the course profiles as also the total number of the faculty.

Faculty turnover for the institute is also very high. The first three batches of students had seen various faces of the faculty that changed very frequently. The institute has been able to attract faculty members with diverse and rich profiles, but retention has been the problem for the institute. The position of chief executive of the institute witnessed similar kinds of frequent changes. The third batch had a retired person with a good teaching and administrative background. The CEO of the institute has been in a position to recruit some members in the faculty with a background of teaching in the best-ranking management institutes in the country. Top management of IMP had sufficient faith in Dr Mad, the director and CEO of the institute till he initiated a war of nerves with Mr Constant, the family representative and regional head of the top management. Dr Mad is a septuagenarian person and highly egoistic. If somebody can satisfy his ego, he is prepared to do anything for that person. Dr Mad thinks that he can read the mind of others and based on his reading of others, he takes the decision. He is also very restless. The moment the decision is taken, he can hardly wait for a longer period to see the actions of the decision. He declares himself as a democrat but behaves and acts like an autocrat.

The student community had a pressing demand for a wider and permanent campus for the institute as the current campus is very small. IMP is running a master's in management programme with two classrooms, two very small-sized rooms called seminar rooms and a small library containing only a few hundred books and a few journals. The government inspecting team is also under the impression that the space is very inadequate. They have warned not to extend permission unless the work on the permanent campus has really started. Arguments towards their endeavours will not help according to the government. They want the increased space properly. The space requirement has been felt by everybody but hardly any action was taken. The basic reason behind the management not initiating the actions towards buying the land and having the campus constructed is the paucity of funds. Cash flow comes mainly from the students' fees. Thus, the supply of money increases with the number of enrolments.

Brainstorming sessions were held to find out how to enhance cash flow. It involved some members of the academic council very actively. Mr Nalaska, a board member, had his own business in communications and systems. Nalaska was interested in getting some people satisfied by giving them some business in IMP. He started taking interest in IMP. Mr Nalaska and Mr Constant were personal friends. Nalaska's idea immediately influenced Mr Constant. Nalaska gave the idea for a cyberage management programme to Mr Constant. The idea was mooted in the academic council. Dr Mad was totally against this proposal. Cyberage management as a concept was just a computer-aided management programme for the IMP students. Finally, it was decided to drop the general (management curricula and to undertake the cyberage programme instead. The entire focus of advertising is now streamlined according to the cyberage management course.

Responses to the advertising were very encouraging. The candidates' turnout was very high. Candidates started arriving in good numbers. They were eager to find out about the following things:

1. Availability of computer terminals
2. Hours available for practising
3. Packages available

The institute had a computer-student ratio of *1:10*, one instructor and only a few old types of software packages. Respondents started pouring in with the things mentioned above in their minds. For a cyberage programme, the normal expectations of computer-student ratio are *1:1* and the latest language programme packages are considered very important. On their visit, the students found a high departure of the actuals from that promised or hinted at in the advertisements. This resulted in only thirty responses out of the 900 enquiries. This makes response around 3–4 per cent. Though IMP conducts a written examination followed by a group test and an interview, the entire process is just an eyewash to show that the process is rigorous. All those who respond are allowed to qualify only on payment of required fees.

This cyberage programme required IMP to recruit faculty staff competent in the specific area. Out of the 10 existing members of the faculty, only one was experienced in the area of computers and cyber knowledge. The existing computer faculty Mr Satwin was not going well with the authorities, particularly Dr Mad. The authority now got a new person, Dr Chouri, for heading the computer department. Dr Chouri was a very bright and upright person. He had developed a very good rapport with Professor Satwin.

In this context, the following results came as soon as the admission process came to the end of its formal closing period

1. Student enrolment is half the sanctioned quota and 20 per cent below last year's level.
2. Because of the higher expectation for the cyberage program, cost pressure became very high.

Before the management, feasible and realistic options were as follows:

1. To find out ways and means to reduce costs.
2. To enhance the revenues.

The first option required further analysis. Reducing costs was possible only in the academic areas. Non-academic involvements are sunk costs and cannot be overlooked. Investments made in the upgrading of computers, the laboratory and other academic infra-structures are absorbed and fixed. This is required for running the new programme with whatever the number of the students. So this cannot be dispensed off. The only option to reduce cost is to get rid of cost burdens on the faculty head. It was further explored and a decision was arrived at to terminate Mr Satwin and get the courses run with Dr Chouri and the visiting faculty to complement and supplement when required. Management resolved to pressurize Mr Satwin to resign on his own.

The other option of increasing the revenue base was also explored. It was found that in order to achieve this target, the institute has to wait until the next batch joins. Thoughts about launching some intermediate programme were mooted. Proposals of launching one-year certificate courses fizzled out due to the lack of funds and lack of confidence.

Dr Mad now rose to the top to throw Mr Satwin away. He adopted his own method of behaving badly with Satwin. Satwin was highly popular among the faculty. A veteran specialist with strong knowledge and expertise, Satwin had also the favour of the faculty. No academic fault was traceable in him. It was decided to harp on administrative watch. Satwin commuted from his suburban residence by local trains. It was just prior to the national general election: a lot of political issues were picked up by different political parties to initiate political movements. Of their different types of agenda, blocking the rails and disturbing traffic movements were very common. Mr Satwin became a victim of this. He could not attend the institute for four consecutive days. Dr Mad started put-ting pressure on Mr Satwin to resign. Satwin had to fall in line in the absence of any protest from the faculty. He resigned. Dr Mad had behaved so badly with Mr Satwin that it hurt the sentiment of Dr Chouri. Though the management of IMP had the strategic calculation to run things by Dr Chouri, the message that reached Dr Chouri was of a different kind. He became suspicious of the intentions of the management of IMP and decided to put in papers. Dr Chouri quickly resigned. His resignation letter was a bitter pill for Dr Mad and the management of IMP.

The aftermath of Dr Chouri's resignation was a continuous reeling of disturbance for the students of IMP, the faculty, and its management. Even after repeated advertisements a replacement faculty with the matching calibre of Dr Chouri was not found. The institute tried to hire the service of a few computer companies for the purpose. Cost-wise things did not match, and the result was mounting student pressure on the CEO and the management. Dr Mad tried to persuade the students to study without systems specialization but failed. A lot of conflicting incidents had risen, leading to the rise of mistrust among the different communities of the institute. Teachers became suspicious of the intentions of the institute, and students got disillusioned. Dr Mad could not escape the heat of the situation. Top management started reviewing the possibility of going for a replacement. Dr Mad was terminated with the full disgrace of the management.

Brief Analysis of the Case of Cyberage Manager

The above case of the Cyberage manager shows the consequences of communications. Dr Mad's way of telling things is rooted in his aggressive egoist personality and selfishness. He wanted to prove his efficiency through the immediate reduction of costs. But the problem arises when the intent is intrinsically bad. For Dr Mad, some amount of patience would have fetched a much better result. He could have waited for some time to yield results, particularly when there is hardly any fault on the part of the faculty. A message targeted at Mr Satwin had its effect on Dr Chouri; Mr Satwin had seen the matter as something impinging on his credibility and integrity. He was accused of something that was not his fault. With no option left, Mr Satwin had to resign from the services of the institute.

It was a real stressful situation for all the operators and concerned people. The message is stressing to the students as the immediate fallout of the two resignations came as a proposal to them for foregoing the options for specializations in the areas of systems and computers. Some of the students had joined the programme due to the specialization offers in the areas of systems. They had even forgone admission offers from institutes with much better acclaims. The case of faculty members has been explained earlier. Ultimately the heat of stress had spread to the CEO Continuance in giving thoughts to a few vital issues like having a wider campus, looking for new CEO and trying to solve the problems of systems specialization remained.

Effects of communication of this sort have been so highly stressful because of the following factors:

1. Dishonest motive
2. Dishonest practice
3. Wrong assessment

Dishonest Motive

It is precisely the conditions and contents of one's mind that gives shape to the contents of the communication. Nicely worded written communication has the power to get through situations on the basis of the intellectual favour of the words. But this is for the short term. In the long term, the motive behind the communication becomes very important. What is the ultimate motive of the communication becomes a very important aspect of one's being, say, for example, someone issues a sweet-worded termination letter for no fault of the person receiving the termination makes more or less the same sense in whatever manner the letters have been worded. Sometimes a bad content with sweet covering may rouse the aggravating sentiments of the person involved.

Interpersonal or group communication becomes stressful with bad intrinsic motives. It is ultimately the motive that proves to be very important. Communication can yield results only when it is based on an honest motive. A dishonest motive will always harm the effects of communication. Stressful situations arise when there is a wide gap between the mind and the mouth.

2 M Principle of Communication

The idea was originally propounded by the current book author R. P. Banerjee in his work *Mother Leadership* (1998). The 2 M principle means the honesty of expression or communication. According to this rule, the mouth should spell out in words only those things that are supported by the mind. It is not only to get support but also to align the mind with the mouth. This means the mouth is in union with the mind. Whatever thoughts arise in the mind, the mouth conveys only that. The dichotomy of one thing means talking of something that suits the context but contravenes the mind. The mouth is one with the mind. The cyberage case has also shown the effects of the dishonest motive of people.

Dishonest Practice

Like dishonest motive, a dishonest practice also makes communication stressful. An organization that is very much into a dishonest practice cannot prove trustworthy through the means of communication if it is involved in a dishonest practice. Rationalizing things into the shape of their expectations would not help. Communications of any kind lead to disturbing or irritating situations when they deviate from honest practice.

Wrong Assessment

Any communique based on the wrong assessment of things is going to hurt those involved in the process. Someone with perceptions of attributes of others has to be the purity and sanctity of perceptions based on the proper understanding of the person or of the thing. Communications based on wrong perceptions are not only disturbing but are stressful too.

The above discussions show a view for stress-free communication. Now, we shall try to present the premise and conditions of stress-free communications.

Non-stressing Communications

According to the concept of *Mother Leadership* (Banerjee 1998), certain things can make communication effective and non-stressing. These are spelled out in terms of the following principles:

1. Principle of integrity
2. Principle of tolerance

3. Principle of commitment
4. Principle of authenticity
5. Principle of head-heart, mouth-mind and oneness

In the light of the original views about the above as given in *Mother Leadership*, the views can be presented as follows:

Principle of Integrity

Integrity is considered as a function of the individual's character, a rather wholesome character. Inculcation and adoption of certain values can lead to the integrity of a person provided he maintains a particular standard of behaviour. This is maintaining a total commitment to truth both in principle and actions. It is attainable through knowledge and understanding of self.

The core self, it is said, is an embodiment or a reflection of the divine within. The individual is nothing but an embodiment of the divine qualities in him. It is the lack of realization of these qualities that make the individual forget the intrinsic or the core self and behave like a petty, mean, small person in their own domain.

As has been mentioned, integrity in character is based on:

1. *Satyam* or truth in principle
2. *Ritam* or truth in action

Truth, in principle, is the truthful conviction of a person who is prepared to deny all except the truth of conviction. Understanding or realization of truth changes with experience. As the realization of truth changes quickly or progressively, the quality of truth in principle changes forthwith. It is the quality of perceptive truth that makes one incline towards initiating actions accordingly. It is often said, 'speak out truth in a desirable manner'. Truth, in its bare form, is the essential one. Any wrapping around it might create a problem of understanding by others and might be deceptive to others also. Through wrapping by covers, the essential truth changes its form and appearance. By nature and definition, truth is impersonal but turns into a personalized form when the covers are there. If a message is true, it should hold good everywhere across the boundaries of space and time. That is why it can be said of faith that presentable truth or pleasurable truth could hint at demeaning truth. In the case of organized bodies, truth in principle could be read as truth as transparency. Corporate transparency reveals both the positive and negative aspects of things that are to be said; it communicates the brighter as well as the darker aspects of the organization. Artificially trying to protect the image of the company through hiding some facts or blurring the facts may mean a short-term gain for it at the cost of the long term. On the other hand, proper and timely sharing of the problems and defects of the company may run the risk of increasing speculations about it in the short run and opens the gateway to the active participation of many towards solving the problems. Trustworthy communications are always truthful. One trusts a trustworthy company, and both are possible when truthfulness is the vehicle of communication. When the organization is in trouble, transparent attitudes could get a host of good suggestions to remedy its problems in the short as well as in the long term. Truthful communications help to generate sympathy. Desirable truth is measured in terms of the ultimate good for everybody. *Ritam* or truth in action takes care of this aspect. It is always better to avoid hurting anybody in the name of telling the truth. Corporate communications can become heartful and yet fulfil corporate objectives. It is keeping to the truth and applying that at the same time. Truth in action thus has two aspects: the concerns for translating the principles into actions and sustaining actions.

Principle of Tolerance

Tolerance plays a very important role in individual and collective lives. Tolerance is an important personal value and can be seen as something that makes the organization look afresh to any problem or interaction through the examination of the context. A person reacting sharply to any kind of situation or interaction loses the chance of getting the full context afresh and being able to take a fresh view of the entire scenario, thereby allowing everybody to take the right position or view for the organization. It is very important for leaders to be tolerant. The other aspect is to take a sharp view and approach about something or incident. A quick and sharp reaction may mean the following:

1. It diminishes the scope and potent of things.
2. It fragments the being of the individual, thereby reducing the scope of the message.
3. An agitated mind might give a set of ignorant reactions, leading to delusion and finally to destruction.
4. It leads to the sacrifices of the long term by the nostalgia for the short term.

Bhagavad Gita says:

> *Krodhat vawati sammoham*
> *Sammohat smritinasham*
> *Smritinashat buddhibhramsham*
> *buddhibhramsyat pranasyati.*

A freehand English rendering of the above hymn means,

> Anger leads to delusion
> delusion to loss of memory
> loss of memory to loss of intelligence
> loss of intelligence leads to destruction.

This network of relationships shows the direct link of anger with delusion, loss of memory, loss of intelligence, and finally to destruction. This means communications at the moments of anger may be suicidal. Any decision or action at the moment of anger, reciprocation or revenge leads to a similar type of thing for the person angry with or deluded with something. Tolerance is the opposite of anger.

Tolerance contributes to stability as it represents the immutable component of existence. He who is tolerant stands the onslaughts of the currents of events. Tolerance reminds us of the purposes of perpetual or eternal existence. A tolerant leader can fight the situation with a long-term view. These qualities are present in the mother leader. A mother leader is tolerant and inclusive. A mother leader tolerates even the intolerant and the arrogant. In the domain of mother, the view of 'exclusion' is excluded and external stimuli are first received, then absorbed or analysed. When the turbulence of the situation settles down, the tolerant leader then takes the decision. Tolerance reduces the scope of getting into a stressful situation. The tolerant person gets into an atmosphere of equanimity. Tolerance reduces the conflicts and potential conflicts, leading to substantial gain in terms of reducing stress. It helps build a stress-free personal as well as corporate environment.

Principle of Commitment

Stressful situations arise with the commitments only towards the individual self. Selfishness pulls the benefits and resources from the side of the organization. An individual who is at the helm of affairs creates a stressful environment or gets into stress the moment he prefers selfishness to the broader concerns.

Commitment is one of the most important operative principles that command trust and respect. While making a statement or using communication, individuals can think of being indifferent to commitment only at the cost of a good corporate climate. It is said 'before making a statement, be sure what you mean by that'.

Unless one means what, one tries to say, all the words prove to be deceiving and counter-productive. The Vedantic belief says of the word as the 'revelation of god'. It is then given a very high level of esteem and provides sanctity to words. One has to be very careful and particular about choosing the words. A wrong choice of words and syllables may jeopardize the very purpose of communication. Words out of the mouth are a definite means of communication through commitment. The principle of commitment makes one true to the words uttered and thereby a greater level of sincerity and seriousness is infused into the context or the scenario. It is said that the process of commitment starts even before words are uttered. Commitment starts at the stage of thoughts. As soon as thoughts spring off, the process of commitment starts. In the ultimate analysis, all commitments are targeted at the individual self. So any violation of the commitment contradicts the principles of integrity. Commitment primarily leads to conformity and trust and ultimately, resulting in a situation of no stress. Commitment breeds a sort of faith in the person or the organization, reducing the elements of agony, anxiety and mistrust. This is one of the surest ways of reducing or containing stress.

Principle of Authenticity

There is an urgent need for the communicator and the communica-tee to be authentic to themselves respectively. By being authentic, one initiates the process of turning the context into being authentic and reliable. An authentic behavioural pattern is a required ele-ment for an authentic system. The process starts with individuals. One individual becomes authentic to him followed by another, making the whole system authentic and thereby the messages passed on or received by them loses their harmful effects

By developing an authentic context, one drives the organiza-tional vehicle for longer. Long-term association between an indi-vidual and the organization normally takes place through developing an authentic paradigm. The process of being authentic is also similar to the process of integrity. These two are interrelated. Authenticity breeds reliability, trust. A person is believed by others when his views are supported by authentic behaviour. Any proclamation of achievement by the company can immediately get the stamp of approval by the employees, the shareholders, the government and other stakeholders provided the proclaimer is known for his authentic behaviour. Mere words of mouth carry far greater weights than heaps of records on papers when people in the interactions are authentic. Authentic behaviour widens the scope and potential of the companies. Unauthentic behaviour reduces the span of control and effectiveness within the group. The final point is character. Authentic communication presupposes an authentic Character.

Authenticity cannot be perceived as a one-time launching vari-able, but rather it has to be an integral component of the character of the individual. One can be authentic always if he or she abides by the divine principles of life. It is the divine principle that puts one on the principles of 'Satyam' and 'Ritam'—the meanings of which have been given earlier.

Authenticity, as we have said, is based on an individual's authentic character as also the corporation's being authentic. This reduces the possibilities of stress both at the specific individual level and at the collective level for the organization. Thus, one can say, authentic communication reduces stress or stops the occurrence of stress both at the personal and organizational levels.

Principles of Head-Heart and Mouth-Mind: The Art of Stress Diversification

Synthesis of impulses and instincts of the head and heart, and mouth and mind also leads to a situation of low stress or stress diversification.

Collective mind and collective sense through cooperation can do a lot to reduce, diversify or contain stress for them personally as well as for the organizations they work in. Cooperation breeds a sense of belongingness and gets more minds to think, more hearts to share the agony and more brains to work out the solutions for reductions and diversifications.

The golden rules of cooperation are spelled out in the Rig Vedas as follows:

Sam gachchaddham,
Sam vadaddham,
Samvo manamsi janatam
Deva bhage yatha purbe
Samjanana Upasate. (x189)

This means that common is your goal, common is your tongue and common is your mind. So, like the ancient gods, having understood the respective responsibilities, one could engage with unified activities and cooperate to achieve the common aims.

Selfish calculations logically lead to selfish communications and selfish attainments. With the involvements or letting in of the heart, the situation changes abruptly; the heart is tuned for emotion, whereas the head calculates strategies and fabricates things. The head is a taskmaster, whereas the heart is caring. The heart always looks towards the self, humane concerns. When thoughts, calculations, strategies or plans of the head are tuned or conveyed through the heart, the result takes a new shape. Actions that emerge out of the situation fit into the holistic design. The holistic view is all inclusive; it has one component that is poised to achieve the target, and the other one considers the sanctity of the means. Purity of means is a required ingredient to the holistic view as well as holistic practices; when the mouth speaks the mind and the heart smooths the head, context becomes caring, compassionate and cooperative, thereby reducing stress.

DEFICIT-ABUNDANCE OF MIND ENERGY

Work-life stress is person-specific. An individual is associated with the means and contents of his personality. A human being is considered the product of hematopoietic stem cells. Man is a psychosomatic entity. The range of acts that man does is based on the dynamics of the mind. Mind energy is considered very important for any kind of action on the part of the human entity. The importance of mind is felt through the understanding of the transactions that you are into. Mind energy is perceived through the attitudes and approaches of interactions. An analysis of the mind would help understand the dynamics of the mind. In order to do so, we shall take cues from some of the latest versions of Western studies of mind and major approaches of the Indian versions. Let us first hear one of the most current studies.

In their nascent work, *The Mind Map Book*, Tony Bruzan and Barry Bruzan (1996, 35) describe the process of locating the mind in the following words:

> When does the human brain first learn to mind map? 'When it is taught', you might reply. The correct answer is, The moment (and perhaps before) it is born!

Consider the way a baby's brain develops, especially the way it learns language. One of the first words babies speak is 'mama'. Why 'mama'? Because mama is the centre of the mind map! From her, the main branches of love, food, warmth, protection, transport and education radiate.

Thus, the baby instinctively mind maps internally from the moment it is born throughout its life, building from each radiant centre, growing branches and networks or association that eventually develop into its adult body of knowledge' (Bruzan 1996, 223).

Mind energy, therefore, can be said to be spontaneous and automatically associated with the existence of the person. Mind energy depends upon the conditions of the person. The emotional integrity of the person is what is needed for the abundance of mental energy.

Mind is said to have different levels. The mind has the power of understanding things as well as the ability to offer emotional views. Indian classification of various states of mind are primarily as follows. Mind consists of four functional divisions:

1. *Chitta* (memory)
2. *Manas* (emotion)
3. *Buddhi* (intellect)
4. *Prajna* (knowledge)

Chitta (Memory)

Chitta is the seat bed of memory. The function of the mind starts with memory. Good or bad, strong or weak, the plight of the mind is first understood through the analysis of the mind. In the personality of a human being, the role of *chitta* is so important that it cannot be set aside. Memory is the container and maintainer of knowledge. Knowledge of things is based upon our level of understanding on the grounds of the past horizons and past learnings. Things that we are going to learn tomorrow are based on the things that we have learnt today. The next generation of learning is based on prior generation of learning. All the past learnings and experiences are stocked in the memory for the next generation of learning. Memory can be both explicit and implicit. Explicit memory accumulates and contains details of the incidents that take place from time to time. Implicit memory does not contain the details but the essential information. Detailed memory takes care of all the steps involved in the process and stores the memory to the minute details. The result of any interaction and learning as well as the process of the interaction and process of learning are stored in the explicit memory. Implicit memory considers certain ranges of vital information as worthy of keeping up and retrieving in the future for the future course of learning. The Indian concept of the style of functioning based on the traits and memory of the past as well as past lives is called 'samskara'. *Chitta* can retrieve the essence of experience and knowledge gathered in this present life as well as that carried forward from the past lives.

In the shorter period, memory stimulates individuals, whereas in the long term, it hardly stimulates directly but the negative effect of this is perceived by the person, sometimes very automatically but accurately. Highlights of the concept of 'samskara' shall explain this point.

Theory of *Samskara*

The theory of *samskara* is based on the understanding of human personality as an empirical self-surviving around the nucleus of a core self. The core self is long-term, eternal and immutable. Bhagavad Gita discusses this theory from the point of view of eternity. One of its main identities, that is, the eternal self having the qualities and attributes, is as follows:

Nainam Chhiddanti Shastrani nainam dahati pabakam,
Na Cha enam Kledayanta apah, no Shoshayati Marutah

The eternal self is called *atman*. By definition, *atman* cannot be cut apart by swords or weapons, it cannot be burnt by fire; it cannot be washed off by water nor can it be blown off by air. *Atman* is eternal, immutable, indivisible, permanent and indestructible. It is also omnipotent, omnipresent and omniscient. There is a specific network of relationships between the *atman* and the human body system. Certain aspects of common interfaces between the body and the *atman* are there. *Atman*, as an eternal entity, takes care of the body till it reaches the culmination. In fact, *atman* undertakes the refuge of a body to perform certain types of roles and functions. Through the ages, *atman* takes up different forms as shown in Figure 6.11. Body expires but *atman* does not. After one body is dead, *atman* takes up another body and passes through the entire process of formation and growth of a life. The trans-life journey of *atman* may have started from the matter through plants, animals and to different types of the human form. *Atman* traverses the trajectory of a few million lives. The *atman* or soul develops through ages in the contents or the quality of contents in the soul. In the soul, the essence of each life lived is caught through building a cord of memory for a permanent sort of reservation. Details of lives lived are not contained in this, but the essential teaching of a life lived is caught through some kind of organic or mnemonic codes. The codes can be retrieved in the future at any point in time for encoding of

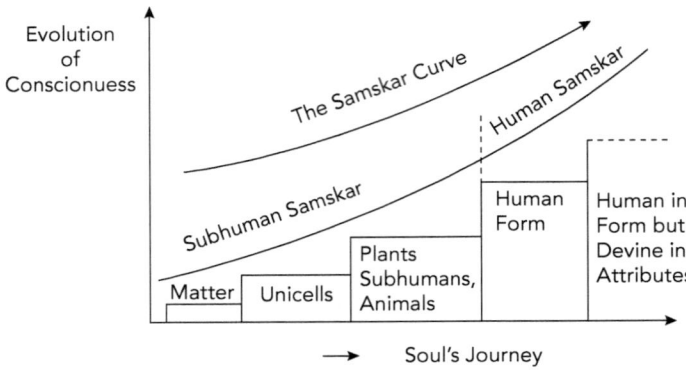

Figure 6.11 Soul's Journey: Evolution of Consciousness Curve

the teaching. Experiences of the different lives lived by the same soul are threaded in the garland of the memory. *Chitta* is by far the total operator of these experiences.

An important point to note about *samskara* is that though it is very difficult to retrieve the memory, it is expressed through the character of the personality. In other words, personalities are based upon the character that is derived from inheritance and also from various levels of special or general types of memory inputs throughout the ages. Whether a person is noble, cruel, holy or has animalistic behaviour depends upon the level of attainment through the living of lives of different forms. Suppose in the life of a subhuman species, one can do good things and develop the intention to rise in consciousness. Forms are direct impediments to the levels of consciousness. This can be expressed in the following Equation 6.1:

$$P = f(C) \qquad (6.1)$$

where P denotes the form the soul takes up in the life of the personality and C indicates the level of consciousness. This means that soul is destined to take up the animal form when the consciousness has grown in intelligence, awareness, attributes and/or qualities of animals. Animalistic qualities like arrogance, aggressive selfishness, Darwinistic propensities, naked hunger, lust and sex consolidate in the consciousness of an animal, and hence, they take up the form of an animal. At any stage of its development, it is the action undertaken by the entity that shapes the course of its future action as also future forms of life and the qualities of life that it is going to live. It is not certain that the journey will remain uniformly forward or upward; it may be otherwise also. Soul's journey is not smooth. From a human form of attainment, it may fall back into subhuman categories as also plant or material categories. Whereas the direction is not certain, consciousness presupposes the support of the being. But the problem arises with the mind of the being. The particular aspect of the mind that deals with this problem is known as 'manas'. *Chitta* carries the *samskara,* but it may or may not unfold the qualities underlying the personality or more precisely in the soul.

Creating Positive *Samskara* to Prevent Stress

As we have seen earlier, *samskara* plays a very vital role in creating a stress-free paradigm for a person. *Samskara* creates a condition congenial to stress-free growth. An individuals' progress along the *samskara* curve is a good indication. If he grows upward along the *samskara* curve, it leads to transcendence in qualities and he is poised toward an integrated personality. The closer he is to the qualities of an integrated personality, the less is stress for him. The individual, thus poised for a superior consciousness, gradually crosses over the domains of stress. On the other hand, any possible downward movement of consciousness leads to more and more fragmentation in the personality and a higher dependence on external objects. More and more dependence on the external exposes the person to a higher degree of stress. An integrated personality is not dependent upon externals. The role of *chitta*, as we perceive, therefore lies in activating the memory codes of positive thoughts, spirits and actions. Thus, it enhances the capacity to cope with stressful situations. Cultivating the *chitta* on positive lines helps strengthen the bearing capacity for stress.

Manas (Mind Proper): Study of *samskara* and *chitta* has shown that a journey could be undertaken with positive aspirations of the consciousness. We have shown that the traits of *samskara* frame the positive of the personality. Mind proper advises the *chitta* to take a positive approach. The result of this network of thoughts, programmes and actions is the gradual process towards attaining a level of stressless personality. This is a dependent function of the acts of the mind. The mind can advise *chitta* to shut its doors or to unleash it at various levels and configurations. The possibilities are as follows:

1. *Manas* advise *chitta* to remain shut off.
2. *Manas* catalyses *chitta* to unfold and unleash the essential experience and knowledge gathered through the living of millions of lives.
3. *Chitta* becomes fully subservient to *manas* and works as the executor of desires of the mind for any kind of revelation and unfoldment.

The three different types of *manas* described above talk of different kinds of situations. Release of full knowledge and experience of *chitta* is possible through the various stages of unfoldment of a personality. A proper synchronization between and among *chitta* and *manas* and the many ramifications of them help them cope with the stress and strains that the person may have. It may be due to the non-functioning of *chitta* in a particular life. A form, a life that the soul undertakes, has the legacy of the experience and knowledge coined by the soul. A positive spirit inherited and coined by *chitta* can go a long way to help a person in the present life to do certain things in a manner most dignified and honourable to him.

Positive traits of *chitta* are taken refuge in by the *manas*. The rate and functioning of *manas* are thus most important in using the information base of *chitta* or diluting the same. *Chitta* has a vast reserve of information base, but it cannot use this reserve unless *manas* is willing to use it. Now the question that remains is when and how does *manas* decide to make use of the information base and how does it unfold and know it.

As we have already discussed in relation to Equation (6.1) (i.e., $P = f(c)$), the form a personality takes up is a dependent function of the consciousness of the personality. An intimate examination of the matter shall prove that the level of consciousness is again a determinant of the levels of qualities of mind. A mind that cares about all affairs can even remain calm, quite unperturbed and equipoised even if it undergoes various stages of stress and strain. Mind is the focal point of consciousness; a human being sometimes feels this and sometimes does not. The mind remains an uncontrollable parameter and instrument with various instincts, inspirations and orientations in it. The propensity of the *manas* towards doing something can go a long way to accomplish things. *Manas'* desire to do something shows that the accomplishment is not far off. *Manas* may have an intense desire to do things. In the presence of an intense desire from *manas*, inspirations for actions flow equivocally and instantaneously. This occurs because *manas* perform the role of a coordinator between the soul's eternal presence and the physical personality of the being.

Manas can lead the personality to various levels of consciousness. Depending upon the inspiration that *manas* gives, a person gets the cooperation from *chitta* and frames his personality. *Manas* can inspire an animal's habit. Then *chitta* supports *manas* with animal instincts or animal qualities. Thus, in this case, the person becomes oriented towards animal qualities. Suppose the inspiration that *manas* gives is that of human conscience to build and work upon; then, related memories and concepts are unleashed by the *chitta*. Aggressively selfish, lustful, revengeful, cruel and people with similar qualities would reflect the behaviour of animal habits which are seldom accepted under human standards. High levels of desire, discontent, utter disgust and aggressive moods are going to act against human standards and norms. This makes one prone to stress.

Manas may transcend its urges. Instead of being constrained by animal qualities, it may involve higher consciousness. Qualities like trust and faith are ones of the like. Trust is a very rare quality in human life. It is said that trust is possible only when both persons have a fairly elevated level of consciousness. Trusting becomes an important impediment in any collection of humans or groups. Arguments could be from the basic functions or factors of the personalities. When does one trust? These are but a few questions that one is supposed to respond to. *Manas* trusts on a certain basis. The universal basis for *manas* is the understanding of man as a divine entity or the embodiment of the divine, trust, cooperation and faith come on this premise.

Manas is the prime centre and the driving force for personality. *Manas* suggests the *chitta* to either remain close-lipped or unleash its contents.

Manas prompts the *chitta* to unfold and unleash its information contents. As has been mentioned, *manas* work on the strength of consciousness. A technical discussion on consciousness shall help understand this concept.

Figure 6.12 shows various aspects of consciousness. The grid divides consciousness into two distinctly different segments. The first segment shows the extent of mind or the human consciousness, whereas the upper segments talk about the divine consciousness or supramind. In the case of the mind, the important things are the ego and the needs of the ego. The mind controls human affairs. With the basis of mind being *chitta*, memory or the seat bed of information rests on it. *Chitta* has been shown as mark (1) in Figure 6.12. The needs of the ego-self are either significantly coloured or shaped by *chitta*. Various schools of thought discuss the types and varieties of needs. The needs and demands of the individual are not the final or even the most important concerns of life. Because of the basic nature or the fundamental urge in him, a human being is likely to fall in love with the eternal identity of his own. The core self provides the eternal identity. It is permanent, indestructible, immutable and immanent. The core self always strives towards joy and bliss. In the temporary realm,

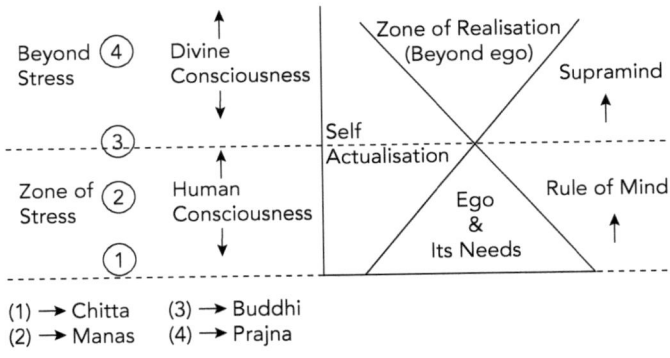

Figure 6.12 The Consciousness Grid

joy stands for bliss. Taking joy in small things is the nature and tendency of a human being. Every element or item of joy breeds the opposite. This means that joy is associated with sorrow. The limit of human consciousness as shown in Figure 6.12 is into ego or ego needs. This span is the zone of stress. Until the mind is transcended and human consciousness transmutes to a superior level of consciousness, a new set of things and inputs to thoughts are the features in this zone. This is the realm of supramind and is beyond the realm and limits of the mind. Supramind does not behave in the normal human way. The basis of its functioning is an overall, holistic outlook and impressions of the sort. Supramind is the natural realm of the divines. It does not encourage or nurture the principle of commerce of give and take. It is a sort of unidirectional thing. Qualities like sacrifice, giving, compassion, cooperation and selflessness are the elements and essential ingredients of the supramind. The human mind is essentially dual in nature; it is restless and turbulent and is dominated by qualities of negative order. It works mostly on the principle of commerce. The Upanishadic reading of the human mind is perhaps one of the most important and appropriately revealing ones. It says:

Human mind is like a monkey bitten by a scorpion which has been made to drink intoxicating liquor and finally a demon entering into it.

The explanation of this runs as follows:

Human mind is restless like monkeys. Memory on which the mind builds its house does not offer the same effect throughout. Now it is here enjoying sweet memories, next moment it is into some sour memories and the third moment it is into tasteless memories. Scorpion represents the sense of burning. It is the constant biting of jealousy. Due to the constant biting of jealousy the mind gets distracted. It is unable to be worthy and fruitful always in all situations because of jealousy. Accepting good of others as good, genuinely appreciating others proves very important. Intoxicating liquor is intoxicating desire. It intoxicates and creates imbalance in the human system. Demon, here, is the symbol of human ego. Demon entering the monkey makes it full of envy. Human personality reaches the summit point of ego. This is the level of self actualisation. Even until this stage as the dominant feature is need, it can be said that expectation denied shall lead to greater ones. It can be said of desire that it never gets fulfilled or satisfied. Satisfaction of desire is momentary or transcient. One lower order desire satisfied means paving the way for a higher order desire. Full and final satisfaction of desire cannot take place. It elevates to higher, and higher levels of demand or desire. Any gap in the fulfilment of the unsatisfied desire causes stress. Stress is therefore evident in the realm of mind which operates oil the principles of commerce or give and take. I do something to somebody because I expect some return from him to square up: Doing something and expecting things on return is based on the principles of commerce. The basis of commercial civilisaition is this basis of give and take. So long as we are within the realm of mind, we are prone to stress because of the longing or expectations from the externals for the exteriorised trend of us.

Transformation starts with the process of realization. Through the process of realization, one attains the level of supramind by transcending the scope of mind. This makes human beings come out of the spells of restricting attributes. They develop equanimity in all situations. At this stage of consciousness, man is above all trials and tribulations. He remains the same in all situations of ups and downs. He becomes indifferent to whatever external stimuli he is into. This is a valid condition for stresslessness. This zone of realization and supramind starts with *buddhi* (intellect) and *prajna* (wisdom)

Manas fails to take the consciousness ahead of it. The process could be a deeper concentration into or consecration to the divine. Through a process of the gradual dissolution of the ego, this can be possible. Ego stands as the barrier to the transformation from the human to the divine consciousness. Work and thoughts can be much brighter, much more penetrative in the realm of the divine consciousness. The egoless man turns into the divine. With this transition, he overcomes purgatory. The situations prevailing in purgatory have been very nicely explained by Dante in his *Divine*

Comedy, a famous classic among the literature of the Western world. Dante Alighieri explains the earthly paradise as the purgatory proper having seven bad values. These are as follows:

The proud

The envious

The wrathful

The slothful

The avaricious and prodigal

The gluttonous

The lustful

These are the various types of sins that humans commit.

Purgatory shows the effect of the causes initiated by those people in their lives. This is a causal network wherein cause and effects are twined in one embrace. Earthly paradise is basically for the human world to reap the effects of human actions based on human consciousness.

It may be worth mentioning at this point that the natural propensity of human consciousness is to grow bad habits and wrong values more eloquently than when a transition takes place in the consciousness upwards. Purgatories are those attributes of human beings that are derivatives of animal qualities. Seven bad values can be grouped on the lines of one value, say love, as follows:

Misdirected love

Deficient love

Excessive love

This classification made by Dante Alighieri assumes that every person is not equally entitled to receive love as a value from some sources. Love should be discriminated against to get its effectiveness in the long run. It is mentioned that pride, envy and wrath are the effects or causes of misdirected love. Pride, envy and wrath are the things that are considered necessary evils by many corporations. Necessary evils give shape to the incidents and transactions of the organization. Deficient love leads to slothful conditions. Sloth features in the cases of deficient love, whereas too much love may lead to lust, gluttony, avaricious and prodigal habits. These qualities are the set of negative ones and need corrections for transformations in the realm of the supramind of the zone of realization.

Purgatories lead to stressful situations. Purgatory or the stages of animal or human consciousness lead to stress. A transition towards divine consciousness is the way out.

Mind energy is positive and plenty for persons achieving divine consciousness. With the abundance of mental energy, one can think of staying above the limits of stressors and strains. The abundance of mental energy is possible only when one lives beyond the impacts of ego. It is the realm of selfless actions. Selfless people, who are by nature cooperative, by habit and character a value based can only do this. The majority who are dominated by egoistic concerns are naturally prone to stress.

This analysis on the basis of consciousness-grid is somewhat similar to the analysis of basic personality types as proposed by Indian Ethos. Personality types can be analysed under the following classifications:

S-type: *sattwa* or good values

R-type: *rajas* or dynamic but bad values

T-type: *tamas* or drowsing and negative values

Purgatories are equivalent to the R-type and T-types. S-type is the elevated and liberating dimension. It is the same as that of divine consciousness. *Sattwa* or divine qualities lead to an equipoise situation and equanimity. An individual is unperturbed by the dynamics of the situation. Happiness and sorrow, health and illness, good and bad, and ups and downs are all taken by him in the same spirit. The prevalent dynamic situations in the R-type are considered an essential quality for other types. *Sattwa* with the dynamism of *rajas* makes one an ideal suit for the organizations. This person is not only dynamic but also remains stress-free throughout.

STRESS MANAGEMENT: MEDICAL AND PSYCHOLOGICAL

Approaches

There is a common view that some amount of stress is probably essential in getting performance or enhancing performance in work life. The Yerkes-Dodson (1908) study was the pioneer in its field to show the relationship in a U-shaped curve showing that until the level of tolerance is reached, performance enhances but falls when the combat tolerance is exceeded. The Yerkes-Dodson experimented with dancing mice and found the result in a U-shaped curve as mentioned. The experimenters concluded by saying that behaviour is susceptible to changes with stimuli of optimal strength, whereas weaker or stronger stimuli had a smaller influence.

In another set of experiments, results of a similar type were found among the military personnel on the battlefield. Swank and Merchand (1946) found this observation in the study of battlefield stress during World War II. Combat efficiency and the stages of combat stress as observed by them are classified into several following types:

1. Phase of battles
2. Phase of maximum efficiency
3. Phase of combat exhaustion

In the first phase, efficiency grows progressively until it reaches a maximum height. The soldiers learn about the dynamics of the battle and adopt them accordingly to suit and respond to the situation proactively.

In the second phase, maximum efficiency is achieved, but in this phase, they fathom reaching the terminal efficiency level. These are recruits who go down hills equally with others having a high-efficiency level but perform through utter exhaustion of the body and mind. The army personnel, in their training, are made to pass through stages of severe stress where the different stages and different kinds of stressors are made familiar to them.

In the third phase, after the levels of highest performance of the soldier, the phase of exhaustion starts. The medical symptoms in the stage of exhaustion are as follows:

Hyperreactivity
Symptoms of anxiety
Sleep loss
Overbreathing
Cardiovascular dysregulation

These symptoms are occasionally confused as neurotic in the absence of an understanding of the causative factors. Stressors under discussion are prone to arouse these kinds of distress in individuals at varying degrees, each being a case, distinctly different from others.

The persistence of the stressors beyond certain limits of toleration might change the health condition altogether. Various factors are responsible for this. The interplay between the initial conditions of the defences and various other factors is important in understanding the degree and quality of health decay. Some of these factors are as follows:

the magnitude of the challenges
rate of the challenges versus the individual's coping skill
the individual's adaptive capacity

Though most of these factors are objective for an individual, for a collective of individuals, these are highly subjective. As the capability varies from person to person, tolerance varies among different individuals. People with a background of grooming in a stressed environment have a higher arousal curve than those without. These people can perform in a stressed condition without generating homeostatic disorders. They are called hardy. Among the army, the Gurkha regiment is considered tough and hardy. They have developed this quality through a successful career of coping and adopting linked with a commitment to the objective. Control over various factors of an individual life can lead to this. Many sociologists have identified two factors for this. The first is the hereditary or the gene factor. The second one is disciplining senses and sex.

Two factors for higher capability are as follows:

1. Heredity-the gene factor.
2. Continence-discipline of senses and sex.

Heredity: The Gene Factor

Genes are the carriers and keepers of the basic traits of a human system. Genes embody encoded information. The process chart for gene function can be given as follows:

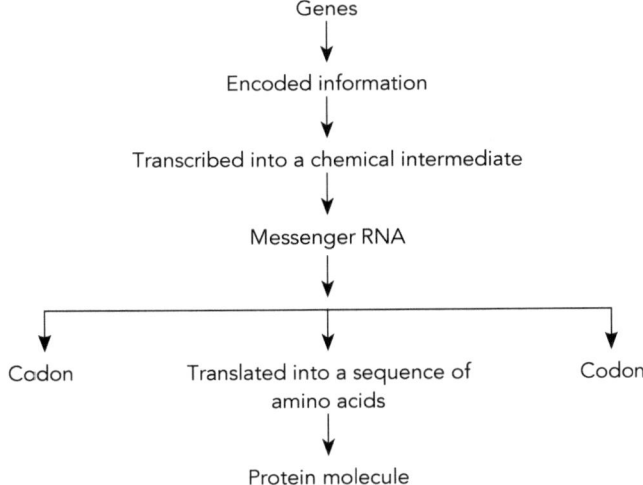

Genes are switched off and on which enables processing and editing of messenger ribonucleic acid (mRNA). Gene sequences contain signals for the cellular machinery, and the information is read out from deoxyribose nucleic acid (DNA). DNA contains hereditary materials. As Edward Yoxen (1983) puts it:

The simplest organism, bacterium, possesses some hundreds of or possibly several thousand genes. That is to say, hundreds of characteristics are encoded genetically to make a copy of the bacterium.

Hundreds of instructions are passed on in the genetic programme to make the next generation. There are even simpler noncellular entities and viruses that may survive with even fewer genes. They survive by hijacking the machinery of those cells infected to make more viruses.

The double helix of DNA in its elegant cellular structure contains the message and quality. The message and quality are then transmitted along the heredity lines. This transmission of qualities in generations normally includes the basic attributes and styles rather than the amorphous ones. This is like transmitting major qualities of a paternal character such as:

1. Strength of the mind
2. Characteristic features
3. Set of likes and dislikes

Strength of mind and other factors developed through endeavours and hard labour are passed to the generations with covert urges increasing every time. Skills are more adequately acquired and adopted for this through enhancement in each occasion and life. The capability of stress increases, thereby making generations more adaptive to situations wider and deeper in terms of generating and managing stress.

Continence

This is again a very important factor in being more capable to handle stressful situations. Unrestrained obligations to sensual demands and sex weaken the spirit and vital energy of human beings. A weak vital is more prone to stress than a strong one. Lust, thus engages the mind towards certain primordial urges, reducing the capacity and scope to fight adverse situations. Rising inefficiency also becomes a difficult thing.

Be it due to specific or non-specific factors, disease symptoms arise when stress crosses certain limits of tolerance. But this cannot be a very general rule. The biomedical model tries to disprove this view by saying that any health disposition is primarily due to the factors that lie and that originate in human systems. The role of the mind is hardly recognized as a significant one. This limitation of the bio-medical model has been highlighted by Gruman and Chesney (1995) as under:

Despite an intense focus in disease mechanisms, biological factors fail to account for wide variations in morbidity and mortality. Moreover biological models are unable to explain complex patterns of medical help-seeking behaviour. Therefore, the only solution drawn from biological models will Fall short of meeting the health needs of the public.

Conceptualizations of health and illness have always recognized the contributions of social psychological, economic and environmental factors to health. What is new is that a critical body of evidence has documented the influence of these factors on morbidity and mortality. The fact is that a group of factors including social isolation, social class and depression predict health outcomes across diseases. It is being widely accepted in the clinical and non-clinical segments of medical science that external factors, environmental social-economic, behavioural and other factors contribute to numerous disease symptoms. Stressors, as they are called, do lead to symptoms of the following diseases:

1. Cardiovascular diseases, especially ischaemic heart disease
2. Hypertension
3. Abdominal symptoms
4. Ageing and non-specific health problems

G. W. Pickering (1955) supported the view that a 'primary pathogenic factor of hypertension and cardiovascular disease was overuse and exhaustion of the normal mechanisms of adaption.' This view has undergone a lot of experiments. J. P. Henry (1975) conducted experiments in animals to investigate whether stressors do play a significant role in creating the pathogenesis for certain diseases or not. Regarding the acute and chronic forms of cardiovascular diseases, he confirmed the hypothesis through his series of studies in animals. J. P. Henry concluded by saying:

It has been established that sustained emotional arousal can accompany the psychological stimulation induced by the social interaction of members of a social group as they compete for desiderata, such as food and water ... this arousal of neuroendocrine response patterns can, in turn, lead to disease states and to a fatal outcome. Various experimental observations in pigs, monkeys, baboons, tree shrews and rodents demonstrate both acute and chronic disturbances of cardiovascular function. These conditions can lead to sudden death or to sustained high blood pressure with arteriosclerotic lesions in the heart and blood vessels. It is shown that when social pressure that has been maintained for a sufficiently long period is relieved, the organism does not revert to normal.

Various models of biophysiological or biopsychological can be developed to see the effects of the externals on the inner realms of the human being. Depressions and exhaustions lead to the disorders or catalyse disorders. This could be schematically shown in a flow process as follows:

Biological Conditions	External Situations	Effects
1. Good health, sound mind	All positive	1 Positive, healthy
2. Good health, ill mind	Contrasting, stressing	Troubled mind with disordered health
3. Bad health, healthy mind	Stressors	Irrecoverable disorders
4. Bad health, ill mind	Stressors	Crashing

The situations described above show the role of stressors. As we have mentioned, vitality plays a very important role in determining whether the person is coping with the situation or not. A sound body and health may go a long way to absorb the effects of stressors and external constraints. Rig Vedas make the following point here:

Abo Udhyagnih Samidha jananam prati
Dhenum ibayatimushasarn Yahava eva pra
Bayam ujihanah pra bhanavah sishrate nakamascha.
(R.V.—II)
As translated by Sri Aurobindo [1998] the above means that strength is awakened by the kindling of the peoples and he fronts the Dawn that comes to him as the Cow that fosters; like mightiness that rushes upward to them expanding lustres, advancing towards the heavenly level.

Through the cultivation of a positive spirit, a man can rise above the effects of onslaughts targeted at him from various directions.

Strength and further cultivation of strength can go a long way to unleash the dormant energy in man. It is this cultivation of dormant energy that makes a man a great performer and achiever. Achievers get things on the strength of their will to overcome the resistances around them.

Twamagone vasupatim vasunamabhi pra mande adhareshu rajana twaya bajam bajayantau jayemahovi shyam pritstutirmatyarnam. (R.V. 4-1)

Strength, master over the lords of substances, towards thee I direct my delight in march of my sacrifices. O King, by thee, increasing thy plenitudes, may we conquer our plenty and overcome the embattled assaults of mortal powers.

As we have mentioned earlier under the gene factor and continence, conserving physical and mental energies prove instrumental in developing capability. Vedas also elaborates on this point urging upon the unleashing of strength to master over substances or matter. Through the invocation of the divine or the divine qualities within the individual, it is possible to unleash the potentials to their maximum height, and the individual then can not only to manage the given stressors but also has mastery over the stressors in their capacities to occupy and contain him. The environmental factors are also influenced or tamed by the presence of superior qualities in the individual. An individual becomes the lord of his works, deeds and fate. Internal human factors prove very important in having this mastery. The belief and realizing of the divine can do a lot to invoke and revoke the spirit in him. Barbara Tuchman (1980) in her studies of the world before the first World War highlights this point; she identified loss of faith in God as one of the deep-rooted reasons behind the evils and ills that men are engrossed in. Barbara writes

...Since the explosion of a generalised belligerent will in the Napoleonic wars, the industrial and scientific revolutions have transformed the world. Man had entered the nineteenth century using his own and animal powers, supplemented by that of wind and water much as he had entered the thirtieth, or for that matter, the first. He entered the twentieth with his capabilities in transportation, communication, production, manufacture and weaponry multiplied a thousand-fold by the energy of machines. Industrial society gave men new power and new scope, while at the same time building up new pressures are prosperity and poverty, in growth of population, and crowding in cities, in antagonism of classes and group, in separation from nature and from satisfaction in individual work. Science gave man, new welfare and new horizons while it took away a belief in God and certainly in a scheme of things he knew. By the time he left the nineteenth century he had as much new unease as ease. (Tuchman 1980)

Barbara has very correctly explained the root cause of our evils and ills. Without faith, individuals are rootless, roaming and whirling into the gyrations of the earth; contradictions and not being able to plant the root of faith in a person can take him on a ride. Lack of faith in God renders us exposed and helpless to the oppressions of the externals experienced through the biological and psychological systems. Some of these factors are as follows:

1. Aggressive anger
2. Anxiety
3. Exhaustion and tension in mind
4. Lack of assertiveness
5. Restlessness and feeling guilty
6. Acceleration and haste
7. Hostility
8. Irritation and impatience
9. Loneliness and isolation

The pace of change that is taking place in the external world makes people unsuitable and unparalleled in their poise in life. The higher the complexity and speed of life, the higher is the incidence of stress. An Individual's divine identity can offer real protection in this field of quick changes. Rene Dubos (1980) has rightly observed that this rapid pace of change is instrumental in increasing the occurrence of cardiovascular diseases.

According to Dubos, profound changes in the way of life, whatever the nature, reduce the resistance of the body and mind to almost any kind of insult. According to him, the increase in population density and the evolution of even more highly competitive habits would produce an increase in the incidence of cardiovascular disease. Kagan and Levis (1974, quoted in Kagan, E and others, 1975) study may be considered as one of the most important studies on this subject. They studied the reactions of various occupational groups to real-life situations at work and found the following effects:

1. Catecholamine production to reach phaeochromocytoma like proportions
2. The level of adrenaline and noradrenaline excretion roughly paralleled the degree of emotional arousal

Nonspecific symptoms create problems first in detecting the illness and then in offering treatments and ameliorations to those problems. P. G. F. Nixon (1993) observed the effects of these nonspecific problems and found how their attitudes created problems for the patients.

According to P. G. F. Nixon, patients attending cardiological clinics without detectable organic diseases are normally regarded as neurotic and unwilling to pull their weight. This particular attitude aggravates the anxiety, anger, frustration and despair that are natural responses to their predicament. For these patients, palliative treatments do not work much, antidepressant drugs do not act, counselling hardly works and cognitive therapy is unlikely to be helpful unless the patient's physical requirements, metabolic needs, etc. are taken into account. Lewis calls this the metabolic disorder or effort syndrome. The following categories and types can be considered as syndromes relevant to the intrinsic factors as follows.

1. Fatigue, muscular weakness and acidotic hyperpnoea
2. Reduction of anaerobic threshold and depletion of alkaline buffering systems
3. Cardiac arrhythmia and chest pain
4. Restlessness
5. Insomnia, anxiety or panic
6. Increased neuronal sensitivity and reactivity, for example, irritability, photophobia, hyperacusis and tinnitus

7. Vasoconstriction or spasm of the cerebral, cardiac or peripheral arteries

8. Increased contractibility of smooth muscle tubes, for example, oesophagus, duodenum, colon and genitourinary tract

9. Hypophosphatemia or depletion of potassium and magnesium

The effects listed under effort syndrome or metabolic disorder are the result of the causes initiated by a host of reasons, the most important of which is emotion. Human emotions are the first casualties of stressful situations. The genesis of heart disease and sudden coronary death is probabilistic and scientific approbation.

Scientific studies of the effects of anger have proved this point. Experiments on animal anger have shown that myocardial ischemia occurs very positively (King and Nixon 1995). They have shown that in man, autonomic disturbance fosters cardiac arrhythmia, coronary vasoconstriction and reduction in the threshold for ventricular fibrillation. These symptoms may originate from the abnormal functioning of the left cerebral hemisphere. In coronary patients, anger can induce left ventricular dysfunction with a reduction of the ejection fraction. It can also trigger cardiac arrest. Sinatra described aortic dissection during suppressed rage. Researchers have shown that anger can induce coronary dysfunction and silent myocardial ischemia. Varrier and Lown's (1984) study showed direct correlations between psychological depression and health hazards. Varrier and Lown observed these effects while studying the relationship between behavioural stress and cardiac arrhythmia, multivessel coronary disease, coronary vasoconstriction and sleep loss. The recovery becomes easier and prompts when the patients are treated for neurophysiological problems rather than just concentrating on the cardiac problems and symptoms. In many cases, psychological distresses lead to death.

Besides cardiac symptoms, abdominal, mental and neural symptoms are in abundance as consequences of stress. The major symptoms of abdominal cause of stress are as follows:

1. Functional gastrointestinal disorders
2. Irritable bowel syndrome

3. Abdominal bloating
4. Functional consumption
5. Functional diarrhoea
6. Functional abdominal pain
7. Levator ani syndrome (high pressure sensation in the rectum)
8. Proctalgia fugax (sudden severe pain in the anal area)
9. Functional biliary pain

Researchers like Almy and Tulin (1947) observed the changes in gastric activity and mucosal appearance in response to psychological and physical stimuli in a patient with a traumatic fistula.

Similar is the situation with the other types of problems. The management of all these is said to lie under medical remedies for the respective problems and issues.

BIBLIOGRAPHY

Almy, T. P., and M. Tulin. 1947. 'Alterations in Colonic Functions in Man Under Stress: Experimental Production of Changes Simulating the "Irritable Colon"'. *Gastroenterology* 8: 166.

Buzan, T.1996. *The Mind Map Book*. Plume: Penguin.

Caves, R. E., and Porter, M. E. 1972. 'Interfirm Profitability Differences'. *The Quarterly Journal of Economics* 91: 667–675.

Daniel, R., and Daniel, P and others 2003. Progranulin Is Expressed in the Placenta, Epidermis, Microvasculature and Brain during Murine Development'. *Developmental Dynamics* 227: 593–599.

Dubos Rene. 1980. 'Optimism'. *The American Scholar*, 151–152.

Gruman, J., and M. Chesney. 1995. 'Introduction for Supporting Ways for Disease'. *Psychosomatic Medicines* 57: 207.

Henry, J. P. 1975. 'The Induction of Acute and Chronic Cardiovascular Disease in Animals by Psychological Stimulation'. *International Journal of Psychiatry in Medicine* 6: 147–158.

Kagan, E., C. L. Soskolne, S. Zwi, S. Hurwitz, G. M. G. Maier, T. Ipp, and A. R. Rabson. 1975. Immunologic Studies in Patient with Recurrent Bronchopulmonary Infections'. *American Review of Respiratory Disease* 111: 441–451.

King, J. C., and P. G. F. Nixon. 1995 'Effects of Non-Right Handedness on Risk for Sudden Death Associated with Coronary Artery Disease'. *The American Journal of Cardiology* 75: 1187.

Nixon, P. G. F. 1993. 'The Grey Area of Effort Syndrome and Hyperventilation: From Thomas Lewis to Today'. *Journal of the Royal Society of Medicine* 81: 563–565.

Pickering, G. W. 1955. *High Blood Pressure*. London: Churchill.

Prigogine, I., and I. Stengers. 1985. *Order Out of Chaos*. London: Flamingo.

Schumacher E.R 1977. *Guide for the Perplexed*. Berlin/Heidelberg: Springer.

Sinatra, S. T., and S. Chawla. 1986. 'Aortic Dissection Associated with Anger, Suppressed Rage, and Acute Emotional Stress'. *Journal of Cardiopulmonary Rehabilitation* 6: 197–199.

Sri Aurobindo. 1998. *The Secret of The Veda, The Complete works of Sri Aurobindo*, Vol. 15. Pondicherry: Sri Aurobindo Ashram Trust.

Swank, R. L., and W. E. Merchand. 1946. 'Combat Neuroses'. *Archives of Neurology and Psychiatry* 55: 236–47.

Tuchman, B. 1980. *The Proud Tower*. London: Macmillan.

Varrier, R. L., and B. Lown. 1984. 'Behavioural Stress and Cardiac Arrythmias'. *Annual Review of Psychology* 46: 155–176.

Yerkes, R. M., and J. D. Dodson. 1908. 'The Relation of Strength of Stimulus to Rapidity of Habit-Formation'. *Journal of Comparative Neurology and Psychiatry* 18: 459–482.

Yoxen, Edward. 1983. *The Gene Business*. New York: Harper & Row Publishers.

CHAPTER 7

MIND TECH

THE WAY TO LIVE STRESS-FREE

The scientific world has learnt to understand things through a series of fragmentations, divisions and subdivisions. Science tries to understand things through fragmentation and dissection until the last divisible units are composed of objects, elements, matter and interactions. Interactions do take place in the phenomenal world, whereas the impetus for and the blueprint of the impetus is structured in the normal world. The scientific reality, which is perceived and acknowledged by doer, takes place in the phenomenal world, whereas philosophies, aesthetics and spirituality lie in the normal world. Issues in the phenomenal world are but the derivatives of those in the normal.

Hegel, a Western philosopher, had one of the most penetrating views about the emergence of man and spirit. Hegel viewed that humans are the culmination of the drives of nature through a continuous and sustained journey of life. Man is nature's fulfilment. Hegel's affirmation of the presence of different levels of hierarchy based on a network of relationships is intriguing. In nature's hierarchy, the attainment of one level of existence is but the function of another. The earlier one is connected to the later one through the present. This point remains inconclusive unless the goal of human existence is clearly understood and deciphered by the realized souls. Sri Aurobindo offers a total perspective that is probably the most comprehensive solution for the future of the universal system. We shall now concentrate upon the truth and views deciphered by Sri Aurobindo. Then we shall discuss some specific tools to experience the emerging truth. The effulgence, universally immutable, is said to lie in individuals as also in all other areas and places surrounding the individual throughout. It is both inside-out and outside-in simultaneously.

DIVINITY IN LIFE

Sri Aurobindo's view primarily focuses on the total divinity of life. The traditional way of looking into life has been in two stages of the development of consciousness. One is the matter and the other one is spirit—the mundane, empirical life culture of the lower self centres around the matter, material gains and material instincts. Total divinity is not a concept but a reality. Nothing can be non-divine. Matter and spirit are the two different aspects of the same divine. The empirical existence can be turned into the existence of the divine. This is possible through the following actions:

1. Total surrender to the divine
2. Unperturbed devotion to the divine

It is the same Brahman that resides in 'me' and the other, that is within and without, that comprises this material body and that which comprises this life. Every particle of existence that contains the divine is full of the divine. Every element, regardless of gross and subtle, comprises the divine. It is divine that resides in everything and the total of every object; every element, ideas, ideals, views and vision are divine. Divine is omnipresent, omniscient and omnipotent. He is formed and formless and can have so many different identities. It is through the sole consecration of Him, total surrender to Him and unperturbed devotion to Him that one can have his presence felt. It is not the traditional way to just see Him or realize Him outside. It is but having the feel of Him always. The existence is the Divine. It is He only who exists and nothing else. He exists in one form or the other. The speaker, the reader, the writer and the listener are but some or the other form of the same omnipotent, the omnipresent and the omniscient. Life can be well lived on the divine principle with total divinity infused in Him. The condition of this transformational realization is but complete dependence on Him and complete identity with Him. If the divine's identity is to be restored, the following things are required in the first place:

1. Initiating the process of total annihilation of the individual ego
2. Allowing the play of truth to its logical culmination

This truth has been spoken eloquently by the Mother of Pondicherry by elaborating Sri Aurobindo's view. Satprem (V-l) quotes Mother as having said:

> Three things of tot3al self-giving to the divine'
> 1. To prostrate oneself at His feet in a surrender of all pride, with a perfect Humility.
> 2. To unfold one's being before Him, to open entirely one's body from head to toe, as opens a book, spreading open one's centres so as to make all their movements visible in a total sincerity that allows nothing to remain hidden.
> 3. To nestle in His arms, to melt in Him in a tender and absolute confidence.

Mother of Pondicherry furthers this view through three formulas. As quoted by Satprem, again, she advocates the following three formulas or any one of them depending upon the situation:

1. May your will be done and not mine
2. As you will, as you will
3. I am yours for eternity

Bhagavad Gita supports this view primarily by hinting at the process and act of knowing the Self and finally by a complete surrender to the divine and forbidding the individual ego. Lord Krishna says:

> *Jnaneyna tu tadjnam yesham nashitam atmanah Tesham adityabat jnanam prakashyati tatparam.* (V-5/ 1 6)

The translation of the above verse by Swami Swarupananda (1956) runs as follows:

But whose ignorance is destroyed by the knowledge of Self-that knowledge of theirs, like the sun, reveals the Supreme (Brahman).

The basic condition of being able to allow divine's will, divine's action and divine's play in individual life is gradual unfoldment through reduction of the selfishness in him until the total annihilation of ego or the empirical self is finally completed. Bhagavad Gita stresses the point of attaining the realization of the Supreme Self for blissful existence.

Bahyashparsh asaktatma bindyati atmani yat sukham Sa Brahma yoga yukta atma sukhamaya akshyam ashnute. (V-5/21)

It can be translated as follows:

With the heart unattached to external objects, he realizes the joy that is in the self. With the heart that is devoted to the meditation of Brahman, he attains undecaying happiness.

This view is further strengthened by saying that the worldly pleasure and happiness are nothing but the creators of all the miseries. Enjoyments are the gifts and endowments of the sense organs. Tested and experienced by the senses, enjoyments give us pleasure through a process of decay of the elan-vital of the body and mind.

Seeking happiness from outside and pleasure and comfort from the externals thus might prove fatal to the individuals as in most of the cases the individual forgets about his real identity, and even if he remembers, he does so as a sort of belief; even though belief is seen vibrant in him, it does not shape in reality. Divine is used as a symbol or an element of belief. Thus, it is an external factor. The pursuer attains liberation from the bondage of pleasure-seeking, happiness-seeking and desire of the ego. Bhagavad Gita says

Yo antah sukhah antararamastatah antarajyotitireva yah Sa Yogi Brahmah nirvanam Brahmabhuti adhigachhati. (V-5/24)

It can be translated as follows:

Whose happiness is within, whose relaxation is within, and whose light is within, that yogi alone, becoming Brahman, gains absolute freedom!

The point underlying *Brahmabhuti* or becoming Brahman is very important. Sri Aurobindo says that nothing but Brahman exists. *Brahmabhuti* then essentially becomes the concept of egoless personality which is fully merged in the divine and therefore acts as the divine. When a person seeks inward transition, a journey within touches upon Him in him. He feels the embodied present in all his elements of existence. The logical culmination of this truth is the all-around presence and profundity of the divine in each particle and cluster of particles of existence. Bhagavad Gita describes his character as

Kamakrodha viyuktanan yatinam yatah chetasham Abhito Brahma nirvanam vartate viditah atmanam. (V-5/26)

It can be translated as follows:

Released from lust and anger, the heart controlled and the self realized, absolute freedom is for such integrated personality both here and forever. At this stage of our discussion, it is worthy and wise again to look into the views, causes and effects of stress in simple terms and then to see how the concept of divinity in life offers the way out.

As we have seen so far, stress is seen as the response of an organism to perceived threats in the physical, social, natural or psychological environments. Of these, social and psychological environments do play a deeper and wider role in the gambit of stress: stress may or may not be real but the effect that is created is of course real

Responses differ at the physical or the psychological levels. At the physical level, the response is unleashing of hormones and enzymes. Endocrine, metabolic and all sorts of fluid secretions are the effects of stress at varied rates and proportions. The adrenaline, endocrine, metabolic and other types of secretions equip the individuals with arsenals to combat the causes and effects of stress. Efficiency to perform and the potentialities to perform enhance because of these secretions. At the psychological level, the response usually creates anxiety, fear, anger, exhaustion, delusion, loss of self-confidence and a lot of other varieties of mental content. Reflexive mechanisms of this sort in nature happen for adaptive growth. Faced with the stressors around, the individual now opts for any of a few ways to respond to the situations as follows:

1. Fight: This is a positive attitude towards stressors. The individual converts stress into a challenge and unleashes the total available energy. Physical and mental resources are used to overcome the stressors. Stressors are nothing but new opportunities before the individual that one must overcome or harness. The entire episode is an experience for the individual, and the person learns to master eventualities in future in a more apt manner.

2. Flight: This happens when the individual finds himself unsuitable for combatting the stressors. He chooses to fly away as he considers the entire thing as a threat to his growth and existence. He puts all his efforts in locating a hideout to safeguard himself. The result is the lack of challenge and desire to overcome that situation. It has all negative effects that occur including a negative growth index for him whereby he tries to find out a narrow tunnel of survival. Learning is missing, and the capability of the individual does not increase.

3. Freeze: Freezing becomes a phenomenon when the stressors are considered overwhelming to the individual. This may be an environmental factor, a highly unusual factor or a totally unknown and unimagined factor where the individual finds it difficult to decide to work upon. This is precisely because the magnitude and scope of the stressor are beyond one's coping resources. During this period, it is natural for the individual to experience a freezing reaction. This phase could be considered as the phase of preparation for the further periods to come and slowly the person organizes himself, amasses energy and resources to combat the stressors or to escape from them through either fight or flight.

Whatever the response of the individual, some learning takes place. Sometimes this learning itself equips the individual with the required energy to combat situations of the sort in the future. In future, something occurring of the sort makes the individual able to combat effectively. If the stress suffered is short-lived and does not go beyond the tolerance limit and is not of a wide magnitude, the individual may succeed in triumphing over it. If the striking stress is severe and prolonged, the individual may succumb to its pressures or onslaughts.

It has been suggested that physiological fortifications are the first-round remedies to stress problems. Other remedies include psychological and clinical. Fluvoxamine is prescribed for certain varieties of acute stress and some long-term effects of acute stress. Repetitive Stress Injury (RSI) is treated effectively by intake of fluvoxamine. There are many other types of remedies, including therapeutic, ayurvedic, medicinal and yoga. Coping with stress becomes spontaneous and natural to a person who is guided by the divine consciousness in him.

Psychotherapy includes two-pronged approaches: as the individual's reaction to any form of stress is based on the individual's threat perception and the energy equation between him and the stressor, effective stress management would involve emphasizing on increasing knowledge and enhancing power.

Whereas increasing knowledge would mean better stock-taking of the situation and assessment, understanding, appraisal and evaluation of the situation, this itself reduces the scope of the stressors, limiting the stress factor to manageable proportions. In order to gain effective knowledge, the individual has to be involved in it and pursue it until the end.

Gaining power may be extrinsic or intrinsic. The extrinsic approach requires one to learn how to absorb, conserve and direct energy to the desired end.

The enhancement process of power includes the physical, behavioural and mental processes. The physical process includes food intake to offset any deficit in the diet and calorie intake. Regulated food and drink, to the optimum level for the person, is advised in such kinds of situations. Wholesome nourishment, developing an atmosphere congenial to good sleep and a situation favourable to pursue life's objectives are also required.

The role of yoga in daily life comes next. Some regulated yoga practice every day helps to relax health and mind. Relaxation and entertainment are essential. Dissipating energy and senseless pursuits of unregulated speech and sex make a person prone to stress. A balanced and regulated life may go a long way to keep up the person's being in arresting stress. These days, psychologists are exploring non-traditional and unexplored ways to tackle stress.

They are not averse to the spiritual dimension of personalities and are exploring solutions from a spiritual point of view. Primarily, the role of willpower is being considered as an important weapon towards achieving that. Unleashed will can go a long way, as understood by empiricists, to contain and tackle stress.

THE ROLE OF WILLPOWER

It remains to be seen how willpower works and what its position is in the divinity in life. Swami Gokulananda (1997) has narrated an example of willpower demonstrated through the power of silence. He has narrated a story from the page of the life of Swami Virajanandaji, known for a very famous work of his, 'Paramartha Prasanga', or towards the Goal: stress gone forever. Bhagavad Gita gives one method to practice. It says:

> Shutting out external objects; steadying the eyes between the eye brows; restricting the even currents of prana and apana inside the nostrils; the sense, the mind, and intellect controlled, with moksha as the supreme goal; freed from desire, fear and anger: such a man of meditation is verily free for ever. (V-5/27–28)

This unleashes the power of the soul potent in the person. It is again a paradigm to fathom the divinity in man. Divine spirit and divine content unleashed continuously, where the divine is felt and expressed throughout, makes a person green and open. This gives him a vast reserve of energy allowing and empowering him to unleash the vastness of the eternal spirit in him and behave like the divine. He embodies the truthful, blissful, conscious and power of the divine. Stressors turn into challenges that can be readily overcome.

The situation that prevails in the modem world among the executors and operators and the immediate physiochemical effects of stress has been explained by many which can be mentioned as.

When stress occurs, our bodies mobilize for one of the three Fs: freeze, fight or flee (the fight-or-flight syndrome). This mobilization includes the following:

1. Dilation of the pupils for maximum visual perception even in darkness.
2. Constriction of the arteries for maximum pressure to pump blood to the heart and other muscles (the heart pumps from one to five gallons of blood per minute).
3. Activation of the adrenal gland for pumping cortisol, which maintains pupil dilation and artery constriction by stimulating the formation of epinephrine and norepinephrine, sensitizing adrenergic receptors, and inhibiting the breakdown of epinephrine and norepinephrine.
4. Enlargement of the vessels of the heart to facilitate the return flow of blood.
5. Metabolism of fat (from fatty cells) and glucose (from the liver) for energy.
6. Constriction of vessels to the skin, kidney and digestive tract shutting down digestion and maximizing readiness for the fight-or-flight syndrome?

All the above-mentioned physiological and other related factors cannot be seen apart from the conditions of the mind. The physiological effects can be seen as partly dominated by the mind and partly by other aspects of the emotions of the being. If the mind is controlled through a process of concentration or meditation, as it is expected to happen, the effect is reversed. The problem demands a thorough discussion of the mind.

The natural poise of the mind is chaos and turbulence. Even a person like Arjuna, who was the greatest hero of the Mahabharata War, describes his mind as being so. It should be noted that Arjuna was the greatest warrior, archer par excellence and the highest achiever. When he was at the crossroad of the Great War as narrated in the epic Mahabharata, he felt bewildered as he was supposed to kill his relatives, the teacher and very honoured superiors in order to win the war. The war that Arjuna was likely to take the leading role in was his destined role to protect righteousness. Arjuna's action was the most important pointer in the gamut of the Mahabharata War. Lord Krishna was himself driving Arjuna's chariot and having a dialogue with him. He was giving his opinion to the concerns and questions of Arjuna. Arjuna pointed out his inability to fathom and cope with things because of his restless mind. He spoke

Chanchalam hi manah Krishna Pramathi balabad driram Tasyah aham nigraham manyae vayorivoh suduskaram. (V-6/34)

This can be translated as follows:

The mind, O Krishna, is restless, turbulent, strong and unyielding; I regard it of quite as hard to achieve its control, like that of the wind.

In answer to this question of Arjuna, Lord Krishna had said the way out was constant practice and renunciation. He urged upon Arjuna for an earnest and repeated attempt to make the mind steady in its unmodified state of pure intelligence by means of constant meditation upon the chosen ideal. This followed by renunciation makes one calm and pure in mind. Renunciation is the freedom from desire for seen or unseen pleasures, achieved by a constant perception of the evil in them. The doubts persist until the lord came out with conclusive words about yoga and its achievements. Lord Krishna says,

Yoginam api sarvesham mad gatah antaratmana Shraddhavana bhajate yo mam sah me yuktatamoh matah. (V-6/47)

This is translated as follows:

Of all yogis, he who with the inner self merged in me, with shraddha devotes himself to me, is considered by me the steadfast.

The way of practice is not even sufficient, as one needs to do the ultimate surrender to the divine with full of love and regard. Consecration unto the divine leads to the full and conclusive attainment of divinity in life. Coming back to the modem view of stress, let us see how this could be established as relevant in the gamut of physio-psycho view of stress

This view of the 'Bhagavad Gita' can be discussed in view of the psycho-activities who have done their studies on the effects of stress and coping. Goldberger and Breznitz (1993) have quoted

Folkman and Lazarus (1988) by stating this. Factor analysis of the coping strategies as given by Folkman and Lazarus are as follows:

1   Social support/direct problem solving, which included items indicating seeking out and use of social support as well as other direct problem-solving actions.
2   Distancing, which involves efforts to detach oneself from the stressful situation
3   Positive focus, which is characterized by an effort to find meaning in experience by focusing on personal growth.
4   Cognitive escape/avoidance, which involves such efforts as wishful thinking.
5   Behavioural escape/avoidance, such as efforts to avoid the situation by eating, drinking, smoking, using drugs or taking medications.

The *Handbook of Stress* offers five different strategies and certain other related actions. Actions do flow from the premise of physiological as well as a psychological view of man. Our approach is quite different. The view of man in the approach being presented here approves the physiological, psychological and behavioural approaches of man. On top of all these views presented, this approach believes in the *Divine Identity of Man*. A human being is:

1. An embodiment of the divine
2. Full of divine potentials
3. Is in a position to unleash the divine potential through strong will and total consecration to the supreme in him

This belief supersedes all other prevailing concepts and beliefs but at the same time contains all other approaches. We have mentioned very frequently at different stages of this work that man is not a needing animal but much superior in consciousness. Man is essentially and potentially divine. It is because of the lack of conviction of our being divine that we behave as needing entities. I would prefer at this point to share a story from the Upanishads. The story runs as follows:

A hungry lioness who was out into the stretches of the woods for food was returning to its den. That day, the lioness was delayed and was hurrying. When it was halfway, she decided to avoid a long stretch which is via a big hill. The short cut which the lioness decided to take has a brook in between. The lioness decided to jump over, forgetting that it was at an advanced stage of carrying.

Immediately after the lioness had given a big jump and reached the other end of the brook, it fell unconscious, gave birth to a lion cub and then died. The whole episode was being observed very keenly by a flock of sheep grazing grass nearby; out of curiosity they came forward, found the dead lioness lying and lion cub struggling to survive. They became compassionate to the lion cub, picked it up and took it to their place. The lion cub was being groomed in the sheep's environment. It grew on their kind of foodstuff and other things; it learnt to graze grass and survive on the greens. This scene of a lion cub growing with the sheep was not noticed by anybody, but its grazing grass with the flock of sheep was seen by a lion from a long distance. The scene was quite surprising to the lion. 'Lion cub, our breed grazing grass', the lion exclaimed and immediately rushed to the lion cub, caught it by the neck and dragged it to a pool of water, telling the cub to see its face and of the lion. The cub did not realize anything. The lion then gave a big roar to convince the cub, but the cub did not realize even that. Now the lion decided to give the cub a taste of blood. It quickly got hold of deer, took away flesh tinged with blood and pushed it inside the mouth of the lion cub. Now, slowly and slowly, the lion cub started responding, coming back to realize its own worth. The lion then took the cub by the side of the ditch to show its own reflection and then said, 'look, you do not belong to the category of the sheep, you belong to my category'. Saying this, the lion gave a big roar to the fullest understanding of the lion cub that it was also a lion.

Our conditions are the same. We hear many diverse views, get confused and start equating ourselves to the needing animals. We reduce our potentials to the small, mean ones and get involved in petty, selfish calculations only. Desire becomes one of the most important tools to live. We live on the lower instincts of life and thereby make ours the fertile ground to seed and cultivate the stressors, Medical science, by all standards, approves or has to approve the fact that disease force can occupy us only when there is a degeneration in the vitals. Our vital force is what we live on and also act on. Lack of faith in the Self is the root cause of all weaknesses. A weak mind cannot cope this stress. The problem is that stressors are given factors or give a boundary to a situation so long as we discuss the issues of stress in individuals. We are not discussing the issues of changing the environments, turning them around and making the situation congenial for us. We are just concentrating on the issues of managing stress at the personal level and if possible, taking it up at the collective level. Here lies the strength of the view we are presenting in this work. The real nature of man is that he is divine. He possesses infinite energy and potential. A strong will to do coupled with total dedication makes it possible. We are familiar with the faces of sins like lust, sloth, gluttony, covetousness, anger, pride, envy. These are all based on the ego identity, 'I am Mr. so and so,' 'I am so special', 'I am defeated wrongly…', 'My views are correct…', '*I am right…'. We always tend to point it out to others and criticize the acts, views and thoughts of others. We have positioned ourselves as the 'best' or the 'ideals', which is, in most cases, false. Self-introspection is missing. That is why we behave like animals and fall prey to stressors. Converting stress to a challenge is possible when we solemnly affirm our identity as divine and nothing else, no less. This affirmation gets us to believe in ourselves and in self-reliance, and we grow into the divine. The face of the divine in man as perceived becomes a face of humanity.

Mind engineering offers a systematic approach towards that.

GROWING INTO DIVINE ENTITY

Mind engineering is the process of making gradual and conclusive changes in the personality through continuously working on the mind. The idea is to cleanse the mind of psychological contaminations. Jealousy, envy, anger, covetousness, lust, gluttony, sloth, etc. are the emotional or psychological impurities of the mind. Mind induces us to behave in a manner we are used to as we allow it to dominate us. This is precise because we think of our ego-self as the ultimate truth. Ego is the basis of our personality and personifications do take place through and on the basis of ego. Ego-centric desires and expectations lead us to psychological deficits where we are being continuously advised to enjoy through the creation of the deficits. 'I want this, I want that'—these wants are poised to satisfy the ego-self. Here we tend to take delight through the urge and drive to satisfy those elements. While engaging the vital energy on fulfilling desires and wants, the mind is deluged with the urge to worship the selfish ego. This reduces the power and strength to cope with the onslaughts of the external environment. Any new initiative to make the personality holistic has to start from thoughts. Mind engineering starts with thoughts:

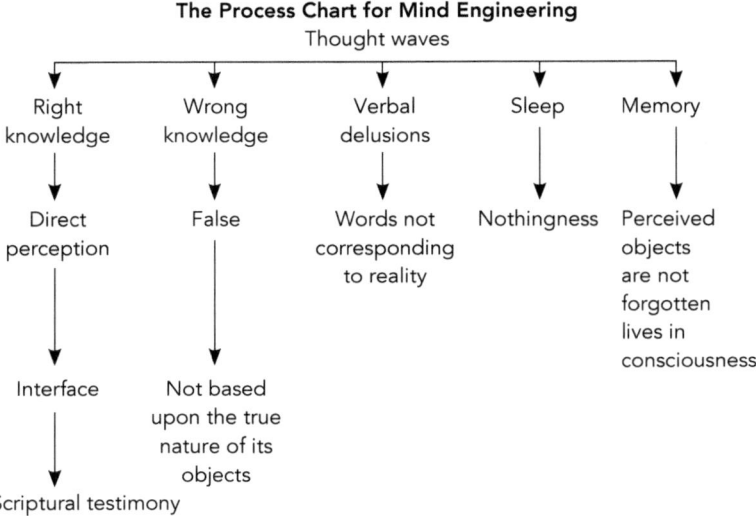

Wrong thought waves can be corrected through practice and nonattachment according to Patanjali, the great psycho-philosopher of India. He says,

> *Abhyasah vairagyabhyam tat nirodhah.* (Patanjali Yogadarshan [1/12])

The wrong thought waves can be controlled through practice and non-attachment.

Practices have to be done for a fairly long period with earnest devotion and without distraction. Practices for self-mastery leads to non-attachment, freedom from desire for what is seen or heard. So long as the ego dominates, it is difficult to attain the state of nonattachment. A firm faith of divinity in the person when repeated continuously takes us to the conditions of non-attachment. This could be done by concentrating upon the formed or formless divine residing in us. Concentration without non-attachment does not transcend the personality. A person has to be attached to and then concentrate upon the divinity in the core self. To concentrate upon the inner divinity, a symbolic entity has to be thought of. This could be thought of as a flame that burns unperturbed inside the cave of the heart, perceived psychologically. Patanjali says five elements are essential for this. According to Patanjali:

Shraddha-virya-smriti-samadhi-prajna-purbak itaresham.
(Patanjali [1/20])

It can be translated as follows:

The concentration of the true spiritual aspirant is attained through faith, energy, recollectedness, absorption and illumination.

'Faith', here means faith in the Self as being divine. When this faith turns genuine, energy automatically flows, and then finally, ego-self is replaced by the superior, divine self. A person then merges his identity with the cosmic reality. Divine acts in and through him, thereby making him convert the impossible into the possible and accomplishable. The success, of course, depends on the vital energy or the 'Will Force' of the person.

The causes of failures as identified by Patanjali (1–30) are as follows:

Sickness
Mental laziness
Doubtful mind
Lack of enthusiasm
Sloth
Craving for sense-pleasure
False perception
Despair in life
Other distractions

There could be certain remedies for each of these. These are cases when one gets medical remedies. There are other issues with behavioural remedies. Each of these remedies is short-lived. Unless the central faith is not restored in the divinity in man, the practices and other things go away. Any despair of not being able to get the concentration shall result in grief, despondency, trembling of the body and irregular breathing. The opposite to this is a calm mind, a still and pure mind. Introspection exercise based on faith in the divinity of the self can do the thing. This process starts within the mind. It works on the consciousness of the individual, progressing through various levels of attainment and finally going beyond the control of the mind. Patanjali (1/33) has offered the idea of cultivating four different social emotions towards attaining mental calmness. **These are as follows:**

Maitri: friendliness toward the happy.

Karuna: compassion for the unhappy.

Mudita: delight in the victory of others

Upeksha: indifference toward the wicked.

When we cultivate friendliness toward the wicked, we get rid of the spell of jealousy, backbiting, etc. *Karuna* or the compassion towards the unhappy make us forget 'rights' approach and reminds us of the duties of life. Compassion demands rising above the personal boundaries of the individual, growing bigger than the life size. Taking delight in the virtuous crashes our pride, envy and anger. Honouring the deserving person is not always easy. People can seldom do that. *Upeksha* or indifference to the wicked is again a great principle. If someone learns to be indifferent to the wicked, he has overcome the animal habits of retaliation.

These emotions if cultivated and practised sincerely make us ready to do the introspection exercise which forms the next stage of mind engineering. At this stage, we proceed to the procedural details of mind concentration (MC). This can be done in the following steps.

Step I: Sitting calmly on the chair (or a squatting position with the spine straight and no leaning in the back. Eyes are closed, and hands are placed on the knees. The person should be dressed in such a fashion as not to restrict the flow of the air inside the body.

Step II: Alternate nostril breathing, slowly and smoothly.

Step III: At this stage, one should allow the mind to settle down at the same posture.

Step IV: Consciousness is taken to the top of the body with the help of willing imagination and allowing the mind to unfold. Imagine a void present inside and an unperturbed flame glowing inside the cave of the heart.

Step V: Back in the original state. Consciousness brought down to the normal ground realities.

Finally, when it comes to concluding this work, we take refuge in pure divinity. Divine embodied in man can cope with stress in the best possible manner and most effectively. This is not for inaction but full actions converting stress into challenge. Introspection exercise is done regularly; additionally, the dedication of mind and consecration unto the divine lead to a holistic personality who develops the power to cope in stressful situations.

BIBLIOGRAPHY

Banerjee, R. P. 1998. *Mother Leadership*. Delhi: A. H. Wheeler & Co.

Gokulananda, Swami. 1997. How to Overcome Mental Tension. Hollywood: Vedanta Press.

Goldberger, L., and S. Breznitz. 1993. *Handbook of Stress: Theoretical and Clinical Aspects*. New York: The Free Press.

Howard. P. J. 1994. *The Owner's Manual for the Brain*. North Carolina: Leornian Press.

Juran, J. M. 1995. *Managerial Breakthrough*. New York: McGraw Hill.

Prabhavananda, Swami, and Christopher Isherwood. 1994. *Patanjali Yoga \ Sutms*. Mylapore, Madras: Sri Ramakrishna Math.

Prigagine, I., and I. Stengers. 1985. *Order Out of Chaos, Man's New Dialogue with Nature*. London: Flamingo.

Satprem. 1981. *Mother's Agenda, Agenda of the Supramental Action upon Earth*, Vols. 1–13. Paris/Mysore: Institute De Rccherches Evolutives/Mira Aditi.

Swarupananda, Swami., Tr. 1956. *Srimad Bhagavad Gita*. Calcutta: Advaita Ashrama.

Vivekananda, Swami. (2005). *Vedanta: Voice of Freedom*, edited by Swarrii Chetanananda. Calcutta: Advaita Ashrama.

CHAPTER 8

EXPLORING
THE MIND

The human mind is one of the most explored entities known to the human society. Yet it remains far from being known properly by an individual or a group of people. The spirit behind the human mind is that of the governing spirit of life. Every individual makes an inch of a journey in life forward with a mind tuned to the purposeful involvement of the mind.

Mind experiences joy, happiness, sorrow, sufferings, shocks and endowments. Thoughts are crafted in our mind to translate them into actions as chosen for. A liberated mind can make many things happen; on the other hand, an obstructed or conditioned mind can make life cripple, restricting the normal flow of the creative or constructive energy into the system spoiling human energy of the earth.

MIND: THE ENTITY BEYOND TOUCH
AND CATCH

The human mind is essentially an entity that is beyond vision, touch, smell, hear and taste. It is neither countable nor measurable. However, we can see the impacts of the mind and sense the impacts through its actions and implications. The mind stands as an independent organ and a coordinator of human thoughts and actions.

MIND: THE DORMANT FLOWER OF LIFE

The human mind resembles a flower that holds the key to all the elements of thoughts and actions of life. The human mind carries the essence of the spirit of life. Whether the mind is in a position to communicate to the external world or not, its role is not only important but central in the realm of life. The mind does the functional coordination that makes human thoughts and actions that can make life free from the impacts of externals. On the other hand,

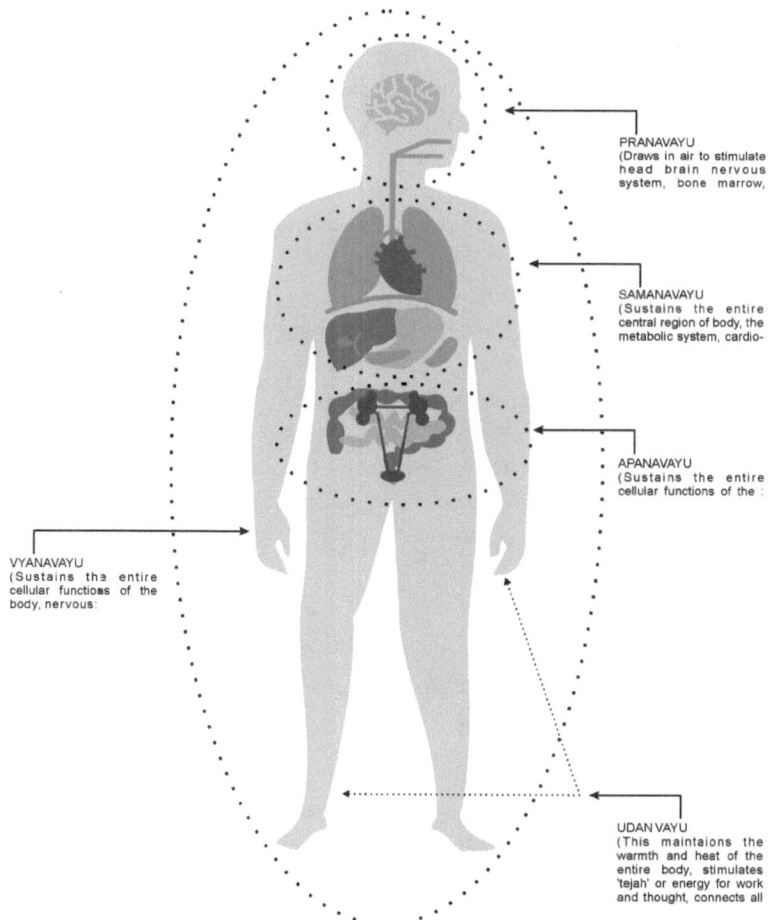

PRANAVAYU
(Draws in air to stimulate head brain nervous system, bone marrow,

SAMANAVAYU
(Sustains the entire central region of body, the metabolic system, cardio-

APANAVAYU
(Sustains the entire cellular functions of the :

VYANAVAYU
(Sustains the entire cellular functions of the body, nervous:

UDANVAYU
(This maintaions the warmth and heat of the entire body, stimulates 'tejah' or energy for work and thought, connects all

Figure 8.1 Identifying the Spiritual Self through Illumined *Pranic* Force

the mind has the option to get swayed by the current events and flow of impacts from the world. However, the mind is expected to identify and focus on the purpose of life. Like a flower, the mind has all the potentials to blossom fully.

THE SPIRITUAL BEING OR THE SCIENCE OF HUMAN SPIRITUALITY

The spiritual being, formless yet comprising a shadow form, made of light remains and resides along with the empirical body. The formless form made of light depicts the essential truth underlying every personality. It does not get revealed unless one follows a sacrificial way to unearth the same. *Pranayama* is one of those tested methods which attempts to open up the dormant spiritual quality and functions undertaken by a person. The concepts of unfoldment go deep into the understanding of the dimensions that are not visible or appear tangible with our organs of senses in the context of the world.

The human organs of senses have the power to see, hear, taste, touch, feel, perceive and think—all these are constrained by the limits of empirical identity. The spiritual process makes it open for the person who has initiated the practice. *Pranayama* makes the gateway to spirituality open. The following fundamental concepts when brought into practice will make the spiritual being unveiled and open for integration into the system of the person. Highlights of the concepts are as follows:

Panchvayu (five kinds so far)

Panchkosha (five folds sheath of spiritual identity)

Satchakra (six plex uses of spiritual realization)

Panchvayu

As narrated above, *Panchvayu* are *prana, apana, vyana, samana* and *udan*. These are the functional identity of the air drawn in from the open air. The normal breathing process feebly covers all functional identities. However, the process of *pranayama* makes it clear, direct and effective to the extent of getting revealed the spiritual self-remaining thereto dormant within. To begin with, the functions of *pranavayu* and *apanavayu* are to make the breathing process continue and happen. In the *pranayama*, when we draw deep inhalation, the volume of air drawn in increases. Thus, this air gets properly distributed

across the physical organs of the body. The functional divisions of *panchvayu* are as follows:

1. ***Pranavayu:*** This involves drawing in and release of the air. This stimulates the upper part of our body—the head, brain, nervous system, bone marrow, vision, hearing, sensing, thinking and activating the central controlling and energizing organ called mind—in different contexts of our living. *Pranavayu*, thus stimulates and maintains the functions of life from a wholesome perspective. With the process of *pranayama* continued for a reasonable period, the functions of organs in the upper part of the body, namely the head, the brain and the sense controlling mind, get coordinated strongly. Thus, the power of mind and power of the entire process of our thinking, conceptualizing, decisions and initiatives for actions get coordinated for enhanced power and scope of each.

2. ***Apanavayu:*** This sustains the lower part of the body. *Apana* helps *pranavayu* in completing the process of breathing through finally absorbing the air within and thereby creating perspective to draw in fresh air again and again. The process of *pranayama* enhances this scope. This helps better in the functional cycle of the kidneys, urinary system, excretory functions and gender-specific biological functions. *Apanavayu* always sustains the organs along and below the naval regions of the body.

3. ***Samanavayu:*** This sustains the entire middle part of the body. The functional scope includes the digestive system, cardiovascular system, cardiac centre, lungs, liver, spleen, gall bladder, stomach, intestine and organs only.

4. ***Vyanavayu:*** This sustains the entire cellular functions of the body, nervous coordination, vascular coordination, coordination with all organs via the nervous system and the vertebral column, endocrine functions and coordination among different psychological functions of the body.

5. **Udanvayu:** This maintains the *teja* or energy level of the entire body. The warmth and heat of the body are very important to maintain a work-thought-dynamism balance of the human system. *Vyanavayu* makes us connect with the entire cosmic system on the one hand and the 'atman' or the pure soul residing within the core of our heart on the other hand.

The span and scope of *panchvayu* become stronger and very clearly effective once the functioning of the human organism is made to streamline for steady progress forward. The journey in life becomes a better one with this *pranayama* having adopted and practiced on a regular basis to unfold the potentials of vital in man. Intense scientific quest is being conducted to understand and catch hold of the effects of this breath coordination process called, *pranayama*. Scientific explorations have considered the human brain as the central focus from where the conditions of mind can be partly understood. The process of breath can impact the brain and stimulate functions that lead to a change of the mental environment, otherwise involved in the process of normal breathing alone.

> While apparently simple functions like pain are showing themselves to be more complex than might be expected, some seemingly imponderable qualities of the mind are starting to look surprisingly mechanistic. Morality, altruism, 'spiritual' and religions experiences, aesthetic appreciation—even love— have generally been thought of as being beyond scientific exploration. (Carter 2010, 12–13).

The mind stands as a messenger in the human system. The mind stands as an invisible organ but coordinates with all biological functions of the human system. The Vedic sages have identified the role of the mind in the human organism. Sage Vaisampayana has presented a conversation between Nachiketa, an aspirant to learn the truth about *atman*, the supreme self and Yama, the lord of death as follows:

> *Atmanam rathitam viddhi Shariram rathameva tu. Buddhim tu sarathim viddhi Manah pragrahameva ca.* (Katha Upanishad, 1/3/3)

(Know for certain that the Supreme Self-called 'Atman' is seated in the chariot of body. The human intellect drives this chariot down the paths of time and the mind acts as the connecting cord between chariot and the connected Supreme soul seated on that chariot.)

Now, the spiritual journey is to make the mind transformed. The process of *pranayama* with its engineered impact on the vital system makes the mind turned to the spirit of the supreme. The characteristic features of the mind would then transform to the elevated mind which is broad and has adopted the qualities of goodness and the spirit of divinity.

Spiritual realization in life occurs through the process of attaining a properly concentrated mind. Mind that is above all types of desires; mind that is free from anger, gluttony, envy, greed, hatred, jealousy and ego-centrism. This mind is liberated enough to understand, maintain and take forward the values of life which are good for society and the world.

The idea of spiritual journey centres around the mind. That is why the purifying mind of the impurities of the system has been the central focus of life. The impurities are the attributes of non-divinity or demonic types. These are actually the common objectives of all methods of realization. *Pranayam* makes it happen.

Annam Brahmahiti byajanat Annyat eva khalu Imani bhutani jayante Annena jatani jibanti Annamprayantiavishambishantiiti. Tatvijnaya. (Taittiriya Upanishad, 3/2/1)

('Anna' or the food for life, or material form of consumption is a form of Brahman. Life emerges out of the consumption of food, and finally, all elements of life converge to one or the other form of food for consumption by some.)

Pranah Brahmaniti byajanat, Pranat eva khaluImani bhutani jayante. Pranena jayanti jibanti Pranam prayantiavishambishantiiti. Tatvijnaya. (Taittiriya Upanishad, 3/3/1)

('Prana' or vital is the form of Brahman.
Life emerges from the cosmic vital existence or 'mahaprana'.
Life converges to the 'mahaprana' at the end of its span.)

Manah Brahmaniti byajanat, Manaso hieva khalu Imanibhutani jayante. Manaso jayanti jibanti Manah prayantiavishambishantiiti. Tatvijnaya. (Taittiriya Upanishad, 3/4/1)

(Mind is the form of Brahman where he is seated. Also mind creates the causative factor for life and continuity. Life converges to the cosmic mind once its span is over.)

Vijnanam Brahmaniti byajanat, Vijnanayat evakhaluImani bhutani jayante. Vijnanena jayanti jibanti Vijnanam prayantiavishambishantiiti. Tatvijnaya. (Taittiriya Upanishad, 3/5/1)

(Wisdom represents Brahman. Lives emerge out of the presence of divine wisdom Life grows on strengths of wisdom. Life converges to the Supreme self and Divine wisdom at the end of its span.)

Anandah Brahmaniti byajanat, Anandyathieva khaluImani bhutani jayante. Anandena jayantiji banti Anandam prayantiavishambishantiiti. Tatvijnaya. (Taittiriya Upanishad, 3/6/1)

(Ananda or Bliss is the form of Brahman. Life emerges, maintains and grows out of the Bliss in life. Life derives its strength to move forward on time on the strength of Bliss. The culmination of life is convergence to the Supreme Bliss also.)

Panchkosha (Five Sheaths)

Scientific understanding of human diversity and human unity has been nicely depicted by the genetic scientists, as mentioned in the post-gene account:

A gene is the basic unit of hereditary information, It carries the information needed to build, maintain and repair organisms. Genes collaborate with other genes, within puts from the environment, with triggers, and with random chance to produce the ultimate for mind function of an organism.

The genetic code is universal. A gene from a blue whale can be inserted into a microscopic bacterium, and it will be deciphered accurately and with nearly perfect fidelity. A corollary; there is nothing particularly special about human genes. (Mukherjee 2016, 480)

The natural position of life is such that differences among human beings are just a small fragment of the potentials of life. The Vedic view of life is the unity of life so much so that every life is the same as each one is directly derived from the Supreme and wholesome. Life is derived from the *mahaprana*—the Supreme cosmic source of the potent of life. The super cosmic system distributes the seeds and elements of individual lives. Every living entity is thus one or the other form. As identified by Vedic sages, the truth about life is whichever life has arisen in this world or the universe, whatever living entities remain on the earth now and whichever living entities in whatever forms are awaited to take seeding and growth on the earth are the revelations of Brahman, the Supreme self. Each form is unique and at the same time each one having derived from the same Supreme as origin is essentially the same or close to the same. Sages of Rig Veda, Sam Veda, Yajur Veda and Atharva Veda have proclaimed unanimously the truth of oneness in creation. A common realization of all great Vedic sages like sage Vashishta, sage Atri, sage Yajnavalka, sage Vaishampayana, sage Jaimini and sage Sumanta have realized the uniqueness of the truth of life as follows:

Yatohvaiimani bhutani jayanteYena jatani jibanti
Tatpranahpravishantiiti. Tat Brahmana Jatah.

So far, the lives that have been generated in this cosmic creation, lives that are awaited to appear in future and all forms of lives that exist now are all derived from the same Supreme Brahma. This means that being originated from the same source, they have commonness and oneness in their existence. They share the same Supreme potential in life.

As understood by the scientists of the identity of life the genealogists represent almost similar kinds of perceptions. Initially put across by Ukrainian-American scientists, Theodosius Dobzhansky and subsequently many others having contributed to further development of the science of the human genome, the genetic similarity among creatures has been tested widely, and it has been concluded that though each person is different from the other, the dissimilarity being close to almost nil or negligible.

The scientific understanding has been summarized by genealogists are follows:

> Variations in genes contribute to variations in features, forms and behaviours. When we use the colloquial terms gene for blue eyes or gene for height, we are really referring to a variation (or allele) that specifies an eye colour or height. These variations constitute an extremely minor position of the genome. They are magnified in our imagination because of cultural, and possibly biological, tendencies that tend to amplify difference. A six-foot man from Denmark and a four-foot man from Dumbo share the same anatomy, physiology and biochemistry. Even the two most extreme human variants—male and female—share 99.688 percent of their genes. (Mukherjee 2016, p. 480). Stem cell biologists and cancer geneticists from the USA discovered, skeletal stem cells and genetic alterations of blood in cancer)

The concept of oneness is perceived only when we can attain that Supreme consciousness through the path of realization of Brahma. The scientific rationale mind has wider tendencies to discriminate and differentiate. General human intent is to harpoon those small factors and issues of differences that are actually trifling from the Holistic perspective of Brahma.

Theory of *panchakosha*, or five sheaths of existence mark, the right position to analyse conditions and general qualities of mind conducive to the growth of the mental perspective of too much differentiation to a close to the oneness of the spirit of existence. Thus, the best-known person and the worst known in the world comprise two states of identities that have close similarities to those which were considered dissimilar before. The theory of *panchakosha* is a matter of realization only. Descriptions in words may not be well communicative; however, they can initiate the realization.

The five sheaths are as follows:

1. *Annamaya kosha:* called material sheath
2. *Pranamaya kosha:* called vital sheath
3. *Manomaya kosha:* called the mental sheath

4. *Vijnanamya kosha:* called the wisdom sheath

5. *Anandamaya kosha:* called the blissful sheath or the supreme soul

Each sheath is a functional coordinating system from the biological, physiological, anatomical and spiritual point of view. The quality of mind keeps on changing with the scope of the functional coordination both at the elemental level and at the system. Brief descriptions of the sheaths are as follows:

1. **Annamaya kosha:** This is the identity of a person across their desires, wants, greed, mental habits influenced by anger, jealousy, envy, covetousness, backbiting, thinking ill of others, evil aspirations, evil thoughts, dishonesty, clinging to untruth and hunger of all kinds.

    A selfish, arrogant mind always looks for personal gains and most of the time ignores the virtue of the world, thereby attempting to progress by all means. Possession of wealth, money and materials does not quench the hunger of the person. The greed continues to glow fire within. A fire to acquire. Anything that this mind attempts to do or does undertake continues to fulfil a part of the sense of deficit but continues to maintain the deficit in a new form.

    Mind driven by the material sheath put a very high degree of emphasis on the factors of difference and discrimination. This mind looks at the world from a negative perspective. Thus, the person carries forward a sense of deprivation. Emotions and sentiments push the understanding that his life is less fulfilling because of factors external to him. These factors would make the person feel his insignificant.

    According to the understanding of the sages of four Vedas—Rig, Sam, Yaju and Atharva—*anna* is food. This is not only the food that we eat for our survival and growth, but this is an endowed blessing of the divine. He is present, invisible, undetectable, inaudible and untraceable in all those elements which we consider as having and in its getting transformed from any form to a new host—the human body. It works at the level of the human body—system. *Panchavayu* acts on different aspects of *anna* to convert this to the energy level of the individual and to form a collective group of them. Thus, the sense of deprivation of the sense of deficit or even the deficit-driven tendencies world disappears from his mind. A new idea of oneness emerges.

2. **Pranamaya kosha** (or the vital or energy sheath): *Prana* or vital provides the energy of life. Energies required for life are infused by the *prana* in combination with *vayu* or air. Out of *panchvayu*, or five air, the *udanvayu* is energy for the life. *Udanvayu* assimilates, stimulates and energizes the entire body system. This becomes further figured when a concentrated mind wishes to move forward the dormant energy in the empirical biological system. *Pranayama* maximizes the energy configuration and release of the patent energy.

Pranamaya kosha is a functional system that maintains the biological energy in life. All human functions require some amount of energy. For example, cardiac functioning needs at least six microvolts for smooth rhythms. The human brain, particularly certain lobes which are responsible for thinking, rational impulse, autonomous actions and actions of contemplation and volition, is propelled by the *pranavayu* in general and *udanvayu*, in particular. *Pranamaya* rejuvenates the mind with *pranayama* generating the process of concentrated consciousness; person finds inspiration to form an ambience of life which actually goes beyond the limits of life. It helps in transcendence of the mortal energy to fulfil and get hold of the touch of cosmic energy in life. The cosmic energy is actually the divine impulse that is present in life. *Pranamaya* thus makes the *pranic* force to focus on the spirit of the divine light.

Manomaya kosha (or the mental sheath): Man has been defined as a mix of the mind and materials of the body—psychosomatic entity. The human form, basically structured around the skeletal of the body we are covered by, is the impact of the seven different structural inputs, called **saptadhatu**. These are bone, bone marrow, blood, semen, skin, muscle and fluid (vascular system).

All these collectively moderate, carry and foster forward the spirit of the living entity. A living entity needs to perform all

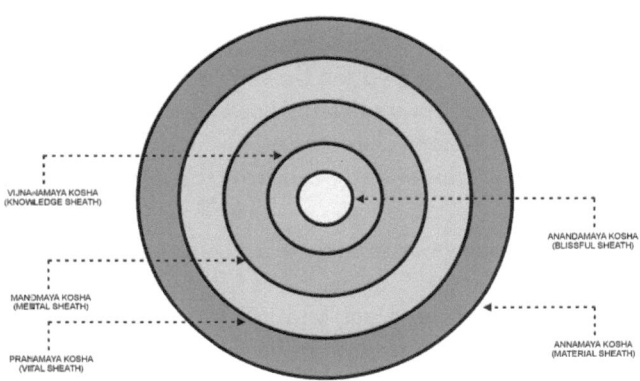

PANCHA KOSHA
[Five Systems of Psycho Physical - Spiritual Entity]

VIJNANAMAYA KOSHA
(KNOWLEDGE SHEATH)

ANANDAMAYA KOSHA
(BLISSFUL SHEATH)

MANOMAYA KOSHA
(MENTAL SHEATH)

ANNAMAYA KOSHA
(MATERIAL SHEATH)

PRANAMAYA KOSHA
(VITAL SHEATH)

biological functions and do activities, generate thoughts, have ideas and make plans and strategies—all are actually coordinated by the mind. The organs of senses can perform only when the mind is added to the respective biological functions. Thus, the eyes cannot see when the mind is withdrawn from the functional focus of vision; the ear can hear only when the mind is into the function of hearing. If the mind is absent, the strongest body fails to apply its strength to any activity. A strong man reduces to an ordinary frail person.

Material functions can be performed independently of any mental support in a mechanistic way. However, the addition of mind makes it vibrant. The mind has superimposing dimensions. Yet, it is the quality of mind that determines the quality of function. The mind is basically restless. The metaphor of monkey nature properly applies to the human mind. Generally, the conditions of mind can be explained in the following ways, with the categories of conditions.

STATES OF MIND

Based on its features, the mind can be classified into four states as mentioned below:

1. *Kshipta* (or restlessness like a monkey nature)
2. *Vikshipta* (or turbulence, monkey bitten by a scorpion)

3. *Ekagra* (or drawn in and concentrated on a point)

4. *Niruddha* (or cessation of mind or liberated state)

On its own habit, mind prefers to remain restless. This is because of its understanding or perception that the world or this nature has denied him of whatever were his due possessions and attainments. A sense of deficit develops, sometimes, not in a conscious manner, but rather in a way that silently captures the mind and acts in an invisible manner.

When the person is confronted with some immediate cause of concern or expectation, it becomes more intensely oriented towards having possessions of those not attained as yet—may be material possession, may be resources, may be money, may be name and fame, may be relative attainment compared to some others and soon.

Restlessness and turbulence of mind are actually controlled and drawn in by the process of *pranayama*. It helps in collecting different forms of elemental presence of mind, scattered here and there, and thereby turn it to the central purpose of life. At this stage, it is the responsibility of the person to identify and fix the purpose of life. The central purpose of life should be somewhat broader and longer than the canvas of life. This broader perspective is actually transcending.

Leader of one's own world has to transcend. The general tendency of a human being is to be one of the 'me too' lot and get swayed by the current of desires and expectations of life. The restlessness of mind shows the fulfilment of any kind and searching or looking for options, ways and means to make good that. Restlessness is because the mind does not feel pleasant at the current state of things and thereby expects many more things to do and possess: material, financial or intangibles. Seeking is begging; however, winning is achieving. A person who wants to become leader of his own should discard seeking or begging. Rather, the person should aim to win or achieve. Winning demands capability building and identification of things those would contribute to the creation of a basis for winning through an honest and fair way.

Independence: Role of the Mind

The human mind creates constraints or liberates the same. *Kshipta* and *vikshipta* state of mind are basically because of the presence of desire, sense of deficit, jealousy, greed, envy and selfishness; essentially human ego drives all these states. The psychologist's view of ego is different. Ego makes one perceive one's dominance, prominence and uniqueness. All these though can be converted to a good quality with the change or transformation of the perspective.

The spiritual process of the journey of consciousness reveals different states of mind at different states of our mind-plexus. Coordination of all these can make mind attain the state of *ekagra* or focused. Finally, the mind should be drawn to a state of *niruddha*. *Ekagra* is a state of affairs where all functional tendencies and propensities are drawn in and around a single point. But the fundamental approach of that is to build a state of mind where the former mind has disappeared and a new mind has taken its position. This is because of the fundamental transformation of the mind. This is the cessation of mind and getting an illuminated golden mind in place. Sage Yajnavalka has identified this mind as *Suvarna Jyotirmaya Manoh*, which means illuminated golden mind, that is, a mind that is free from clutches of desires, deficits, greed, anger, lust, discrimination, hatred, gluttony and covetousness and hunger for possession of money-material-fame and devoid of personal ego.

1. **Vijnanamya kosha** (or the wisdom sheath): Knowledge can be acquired, but wisdom is present within every individual. It just awaits surfacing up. Unleashing of intrinsic content of knowledge, understanding, perception, realization or acquired inputs of learning together along with other inputs from the outside environment or the world makes it vibrant to reveal the factors of wisdom for the quest of truth in life. Knowledge forms the external layer of wisdom. Knowledge takes into cognizance the spirit of work, the work energy and the required inspiration for accomplishing the work. *Vijnana* is that special variety of work that contributes the wholesome perspective, the context of work, the objective of work and finally the resultant drive that the work contributes to. *Vijnanamya* thus embraces the entire stream of work, thoughts behind the work and the resultant effect of the work.

   Vijnanamya state of consciousness makes the gateway to wisdom open and transform lives to the extent of making the mind think good of all. Vedic sages have unanimously described the basic objective of this state of mind as: *Sarve Bhavantu Sukhinah, Sarve Santu Niramaya* (or let everyone become happy. Let the well-being gets distributed to all). This mind does not depend on any material advantages or gains, rather the mind wants that all be good and happy for all. Wisdom breeds in when the person is free from impacts of ego.

2. *Anandamaya kosha* (or the blissful sheath): Whereas the wisdom sheath has still the causes for differentiation when the consciousness touches the core of our existence, it finds the vast pool of blissful condition and gets immersed in from the spiritual view of understanding. The human being is considered to have three different forms from a mix of empirical and spiritual understanding. These are the material body, the subtle body and the causal body. The material body is the physical body as we understand it from the rational-physical and biological perspective. The material body has been profusely described in various ways through biological sciences, branches of medical sciences-anatomical, physiological and anthropological descriptions. Also, human existence has been described in environmental, social and other ways. The material body, though material in its form and appearance, has still proved impenetrable in terms of the knowledge of the system of the material body. The mind is the central organ that coordinates and controls everything of the physical body. Some scientists assume the seat of the mind is the human brain. However, the spiritual analysis identifies that the mind resides at all seven-spiritual plexus with seven different identities. Attempts to map the contents and activities of the human brain have shown and proved that our knowledge and capacity touch only about a part of several million segments of a grown brain organ. One of the most prominent scientific understandings of the human brain as depicted by neuroscientists maintains that:

In normal brains incoming sensory stimuli follow well-worn neutral paths from the sensory organ to specific brain destinations. As the stimulus passes through the brain it is split into several different streams which are processed in parallel by different brain modules. Some of these modules are in the cerebral context..., others are in the limbic system. Every brain constructs the world in a slightly different way from any other because every brain is different. The sight of an external object will vary from person to person because no two people have precisely the same number of motion cells, magneta-sensitive cells, or straight-line cells... An individual view is formed both by their genes and by how their brain has been modulated by experience. (Carter 2010, 175–178)

The scientific analysis of the brain shows and depicts the difference in the biological composition of the brain to an extent that is a very small segment of it. Most part and functional tendencies are the same. Thus, the difference between a good man and that of a bad man is very small and can be removed gradually. This difference can be made good through efforts of the kind of *pranayama*. With the effective control of this act and practice of *pranayama*, the person gets the *pranic* forced stimulated forward so much so that the goodness of habit and character gets revealed on the one hand and the creative faculty of the person gets unfolded on the other hand. As has been mentioned by the latest idea of neuroscience, our consciousness gets stimulated on a positive scale either as a result of its genealogical positions or through the experience earned in life. A person is considered divinely if he has all the good qualities as has been spelled before. A spiritual seeker would develop set qualities that are divine. He should be a person full of simplicity like an ordinary child—mild, modest, honest, sincere and sweet in his words—has a unique level of consciousness of a noble being and at the same time realizes the identity of own self and sees the same self everywhere—perceives oneness with all and thereby bears in mind that the same Supreme, the Brahmana, resides in all personalities, the same way as it is present in him. At the level of *pranayama* getting intents vigorously, the vital energy within which micro-cosmic gets in touch with or connects with the outer, the micro-cosmic.

With the connection between the micro-cosmic and the acro-cosmic, the super cosmic union occurs and the realization of Supreme, the Brahma occurs, and thus the consciousness attains the highest abode, known as the divine plexus or *Sahasrara*. The communion makes life blissful, *ananadamaya,* where the person who is aspirant of spiritual attainment gets merged in the godly bliss in life. *Brahmavid Brahmaiva Vavati* implies that the realized person has realized the spirit of Brahma and has attained the spirit of Brahma.

Shatchakra (Six Spiritual Plexus)

The spiritual attainment happens in the course of our experience of the journey of consciousness and in the process having gradual transformation of the consciousness from the usual human attributes to divine identity of a person.

The spiritual identity of a person and gradual experience are stored in the consciousness. This gets revealed to the person who has actually initiated and adopted actively into the process. Realization is actually self-experiencing and self-discovery. This is a continuous process. The plexus acts at six different points and connects this body with the invisible inner dimension. The inner dimensions are viewed from the following angles:

- Physical material body
- The subtle body
- The causal body

Spiritual realizations occur at the level of the subtle body -which is an invisible existence remaining present within the current existence. The causal body contemplates, delivers and fosters the acquired experience and translates the earned experience into the wisdom of life. The main messenger of spiritual impulse is the set of pathways that have a built-in presence in human existence. The channels which contain, transmit and helps in transforming are subtle yet empirical.

In the composition of the human body, we have the following:

- *SUSUMNA* (this refers to the notochord—the vertebral column that runs from the tail end of the vertebral column, leading up to the skull. Bone marrow of the central column runs through the vertebral column).
- *IDA* (this is a channel that runs from the base of *susumna* and turns left to *susumna* up to the upper end of the throat level and converges to the left nostril).

- *PINGALA* (this is a channel that runs right of the *susumna*, the central column and runs up to the upper end of the throat level and converges to the right nostril).

The *chakras* or plexus are as follows:

Muladhara: or the root *chakra* is located at the tail end of the spinal column. The consciousness of the human self rests here in the form of a serpent that has three and a half coils. This is in a sleeping state. The purpose of an aspirant in a spiritual journey is to invoke the conscious form—sleeping in the form of a serpent. This self is the seat bed of Shakti—the primordial energy and the energy released by the *pranic* forces reveal the condition for the arousal of the coiled spirit. With invocation, the coil starts unfolding and ultimately this indicates movement upward through the spinal column of *susumna*. A storehouse of biological and spiritual energy, *muladhara* opens its flow through the channel of *susumna* with the touch of the *pranavayu* in general and *apanavayu* in particular.

The action of *apanavayu* ranges from the naval region to below. It connects the physiological functions of the entire excretory process, the kidneys and regions or functions supporting it and associated with it. Also, this *apanavayu* has a direct action on the genitals and the entire related functions. The mental habit of lower instincts and various varieties of lower properties can be coordinated and controlled through the process of *pranayama*.

The channels or *nadis* of *ida* and *pingala* are connected through alternate nostril breathing. *Ida* is governed through the left nostril, whereas that of *pingala* through the right nostril. The serpents that stay almost sleepy at the base of *susumna* at *muladhara*, block the *susumna* channel fully. *Ida* and *pingala* make the first crossover at this point. When a spiritual aspirant is into the process of alternate nostril breathing, air inhaled passes through either of them, reaches the lowermost channel and exchanges its pathway of passage. *Ida* is considered as feminine in nature and taken as lunar in character, whereas the other one *pingala* is considered as masculine in nature and is considered as Sun in life. For effective utilization of the functioning of alternate nostril breathing, it is suggested that the process be initiated with the *pranicvayu* (drawn from atmosphere) and drawn through the right nostril first while keeping the left nostril closed. Repetition of the process would enable the person carry the *pranicvayu* drawn through the right nostril down to the level of *muladhara*. The *pranicvayu* splits in five characters, as mentioned before, as follows.

Pranavayu: It covers the areas above the throat level.

Apanavayu: It goes down to naval region and entire position below.

Samanavayu: It covers the regions below throat up to the naval region.

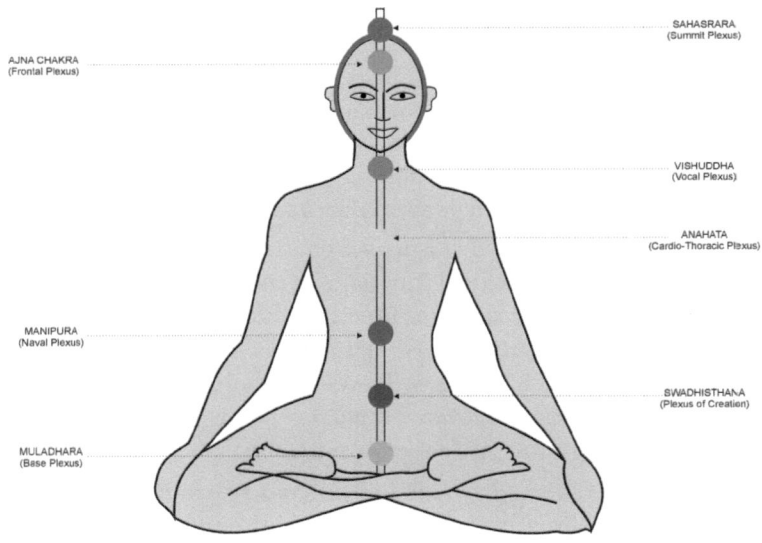

Yanavayu: It covers the entire endocrine, nervous system and vascular systems.

Udanvayu: It generates and distributes energy (vital) to all cells.

Thus, it remains with the *apanavayu* to take care of the regions at *muladhara*. The *pingala* channel opens up gradually, with the movement of *apanavayu* downwards, up to the junction at *muladhara*. Sufficient flow of this with the mind properly attached to it makes the *pranicvayu* reach the lower most end of the *pingala*. Now is the time to stimulate the serpent of *shakti* (energy—at the primordial state) to awaken and raise its head forward, releasing the *pranic* air through *ida*, up to the left nostril, to be released in open air, on the one hand, and the *susumna* to gradually move upwards with all its contents. The process does not occur just as it is. It requires sustained practice, mental attention and total devotion. Once the journey of the *susumna* is completed, it makes the energy flow meet at different levels of plexus with different objectives. The visual effects of a teach plexus are different.

Ida and *pingala* do crossover at certain points. It is like two or three rivers joining with each other and flowing up or down thereafter, like the presence of *Triveni* (three streams)—rivers such as the Ganges, Yamuna and Saraswati meeting at the crossover, each of which is a plexus. These plexuses are named as: *muladhara* (1), *svadhisthana* (2), *manipura* (3), *anahata* (4), *vishuddha* (5), *ajnaa* (6) and *sahasrara* (7). This central column starts with *muladhara* and ends up with *susumna*.

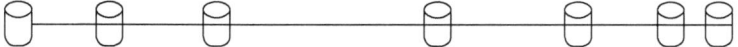

(The vertical column with 1 as the basement is shown here horizontally.)

The descriptions about plexuses are actually subjective. This spiritual process is experiential. Experiences attained by a seeker in this journey are unique to the persons. However, certain things, in general, will be in common with everyone. Certain visuals like lotus with differential colours and number of petals viewed in most cases are briefly mentioned here. The basic nature of each of the plexuses has common understanding.

1. ***Muladhara:*** This is situated at the base of the spinal column at the sacral or pelvic plexus as one understands while in medication. The colours appear red revealed through clear or somewhat depiction of a lotus with four petals. *Muladhara* is actually the base plexus. It is considered as the storehouse of all physical, mental and spiritual energies for empirical and spiritual functions. *Chitta—Manas*—these two states of mind reside here. *Chitta* is the seat bed of memory, and *manas* is the thinking organ of mind. *Muladhara* is considered to have elephantine nature—profuse energy, but reserved. The form of an elephant carrying four-petalled lotus is meaningful here. Four petals represent the four different goals of

life—*dharma, artha, kama* and *moksha*—*dharma* is righteousness, *artha* stands for the meaning of life established through possessions, or maybe giving up, in some rare cases. The possessions could be material, money, resources, fame, establishments, etc., of various nature. *Kama* refers to desires. It means fulfilling desires of any kind. Usually, this refers to the desires for instincts lower in nature is actually meant by it. *Moksha* refers to liberation. It is defined as liberation from all kinds of material bondages. *Moksha* is the spiritual attainment in achieving the wisdom of supreme self-'Brahman'.

Persons who have a dominant intent to enjoy life and who are deluged with the enjoyments of material nature would always get their consciousness bonded down and move within the limits of the first three plexuses—*muladhara, svadhisthana* and *manipura*. However, the other few individuals who intend to have superior quality of life are able to transcend the barriers of *manipura* and move upward while intending to reach the top—the seventh plexus called *sahasrara*.

All the levels of *muladhara*, that is, the quality of mind, is such that all non-divine qualities—such as greed, anger, jealousy, lust, covetousness, envy, loath, untruth and evil mind—become the basic make-up of mind. Mind, at this level, is dominated by selfish tendencies and always carry the message of selfish gains, that too at any cost. The mental drive being non-divine, the condition at *muladhara* is such that the governance of life is exteriorized or externally oriented. With the mind drawing inputs from the external—the *muladhara* mind is utterly selfish and evil thinker. This mind propels a person to do whatever offers a personal gain to them at any cost. Mind at *muladhara* is basically dominated by ego of the person. Ego is revealed through selfishness, greed, desire and tendencies, which are considered to be low in nature. People with this type of nature can do any kind of evil work and can always think evil. This mind can also be opened up with spiritual process, even if it is imposed on the person.

2. *Svadhisthana* **(or one's own place—the origin of birth and creations):** This has a reference of being based at the vertebral column located at the place of genitals in the lower part of lower abdomen. Biological position can be further estimated to lie

between the coccyx and sacrum. Its colour is the colour of fire. This level shows a lot of activities—joy, happiness, hope, self-confidence driven by either the positive spiritual energy or by a neutral biologically driven energy. *Svadhisthana*—considered as the own place—makes the general motive of work vibrant. With *pranic* energy added to the subconscious also joins the process of change and transformation at the level of *svadhisthana chakra*. This plexus requires direct control through the impetus of the *sushumna*. As the *sushumna* wave rises, our intent at this plexus purifies. Getting washed off the impurities at this stage, at the *svadhisthana* level, understanding of the spiritual intent develops and thereby the urge for the lower instincts and desires that are primordial in nature do diminish gradually, allowing the noble intent of life to grow deeper and larger. This life force helps in activating the flower of life blossoming into its full potential. The person, thus, reaches the height of purity but is guided by the vehicle of dynamism to cover all activities of life in one place.

Svadhisthana plexus is, thus, a very important point in the spiritual journey of a man. *Ida* and *pingala*—who are logically the masters of feminine attributes and masculine attributes—do cross-over and meet at the level of the *muladhara* at a higher plane. So *svadhisthana* gets the *sushumna* flow through this plexus and the *pranic* force through the *pranavayu*. *Svadhisthana* chakra has six petals of vermillion coloured lotus. These six petals of lotus represent six attributes of vices—*kama* (desire), *krodha* (anger), *lobha* (greed), *moha* (delusions), *mada* (jealousy/addicted) and *matsarya* (chaotic)—are attributes that lead to create a personality negative to the progress of spiritual energy. That is why these attributes are considered as being enemies to a spiritual aspirant. These are the attributes that collectively and singularly create an obstacle to the progress of the person.

The *pranic* force, which is associated with vital energy, remains at *svadhisthana* and can create wonder. One who can overcome the impacts of these negative attributes attains the strength to move fast and forward. *Svadhisthana* creates the pathway or destroys it. One who falls prey to or gets attracted to the allurements of the enjoyment of this plexus gets kicked off from the pathways of inner spirituality. The inner spirituality has to be rejuvenated through avoidance and rejection of the vices or the six negative elemental attributes. Thus, *svadhisthana* helps the process to attain goodness and divine attributes in life for a spiritual seeker.

3. **Manipura** (or the naval plexus): This plexus is known as the solar plexus. *Manipura* is the centre through which the journey of life continues. At the level of gradual formation within the being of the mother, the entire vital energy is used to get infused into the new life through the naval cord. Once it is cut apart at the naval root, the naval cord remains a very important plexus for the continuity of the genealogical factors. The *manipura* plexus is actually a transitional junction between the material orientation of life and the spiritual orientation of life. A naval plexus is a place where one can get the light of life. The question that can be asked is what kind of life does the person prefer to choose from. If the dominant intent of life is to seek material comfort, biological pleasure, social recognition in terms of name and fame, he can finally create a relative position of advantage in terms of gains in life. *Muladhara* is a plane where the human consciousness may reflect back and move down to *svadhisthana* and *muladhara*. This occurs in most of the cases. However, if by means of any inspiration, motivation or sensitization, the human mind develops attraction towards spiritual path, it paves open the journey of spiritual energy throughout the *sushumna* column. With mind opened to the spiritual path, the upward passage of spiritual energy is initiated. This moves towards the next higher plexus, called *anahata* (throat *chakra*). All conditions being conducive to spiritual journey, the conscious energy meets the plexus at the centre of the throat and merges with the elemental consciousness. At this level, the spiritual aspirant visualizes 10 petalled lotus—these represent the *dasa mahavidya* or 10 great spirits. These are forms of goddess Kali. The *dasa mahavidya* are the different forms of appearance of the supreme mother, Mahadevi Durga. The forms are as follows: Mahakali, Tara, Bhairavi, Chhinnamasta, Chandi, Bhubaneswari, Bagala, Kamala, Katyayani and Durga. All these are different revelations of the same supreme mother, Durga (also named as Devi Parvati, Devi Vaishnavi, etc.). Depending on the condition of the mind of aspirants, the form of the devi appears in realization, which is appropriate to him.

The *manipura* plexus is actually like a city of jewels. It has so many parts and other precious elements. When the elemental value of the plexus is made, the direction and quality of movement of the spiritual energy is important. Wisdom, rationality, emotions, principles, values and concerns, all are contained at this level. When the journey upward is permitted, all these qualities set more finely. On the other hand, if the spiritual energy is reflected to the downward level, the attributes that dominate the person are opposite in nature.

At the level of *manipura* plexus the *ida* and *pingala* crossover. So the *pranic* forces meet there, carried by *samanavayu*. Known otherwise as the fire of life, it helps in metabolism and digestion and helps in functioning of organs in the pelvic region and the abdominal region—major organs in the abdomen and the lower regions are facilitated by the fire that is stored and generated at the naval region. They also help in maintaining the physiological balance across the diaphragm.

The spiritual idea about crossing over this level at the naval region is purely an experiential effort. Being mostly subjective in nature, *manipurachakra* offers the power and energy to transform the individual experience to a collective understanding through collective consciousness.

Awakening of our spiritual self occurs at *manipura*, first, and gradually the same gets added impetus from the subsequent plexuses through meditation.

4. **Anahata** (or the cardiac centre): *Anahata* means unhurt. It lies at the cardiac region within the central spinal column. Comprising 12 petals, the lotus at this *anahata* plexus has the colour of the sky and invites the openness of the vast universe and the atmosphere. *Anahata* is symbolized as two inverted triangles, one of which points upward and the other points downwards. Even at this level, the spiritual aspirant may get attracted by the lowness of life—which is depicted by showing the lower-directed triangle. The triangle that points upward indicates the journey of our consciousness upward. This connects with the cosmic system. *Anahata* plexus generates goodness of life. It allows us to experience the goodness of the cosmic system. The vast presence of the supreme being opens the door of experience here.

Anahata plexus vibrates with the super cosmic original sound of 'OM' pronounced as 'O-U-M' in a rhythm. This unheard sound is actually soundless sound that helps elevate our mind towards *bhuma* (the cosmic whole). Once the sensitization of *bhuma* is achieved, the cosmic wholeness touches our cardiac centre, and we begin the journey in *bhakti* or devotion to god. The meditation at *anahatachakra* helps one to be devoted. However, a concentrated mind may fall down and instead of moving upward, the consciousness of the aspirant may consider the empirical. Material identity is more attractive. Thus, the aesthetic view and emotions come into focus. The aspirant, in this case, considers the material context of love and happiness. The aspirant also finds this clearly dear and thereby considers this to be the essential truth in life. At this level, those 12 petals represent 9 stages of devotion, called *nababidhabhakti*, and three stages of energy, called *trayeeshakti*. The bhakti elements are as follows: *shravana, kirtana, Vishnu smarana, padasevana, archana, vandana, dasya, sakhya, aatmanivedana* or hearing of godly message, chanting, remembering god, service to lord, offerings, dedicating spirit, gods, servanthood, friendhood and self-concentration. However, the *trayeeshakti* refers to *kriyashakti, gunashakti* and *jnanashakti*— or the energy for dedicated work, the values divinely in character and wisdom—knowledge of god.

This cardiac plexus allows the unfolding of the realization of Supreme in one and the absolute, the infinite. This is termed as *bhuma*.

> *Yoh vai Bhuma tatsukham, Nahalpe sukhamasti, Bhumaeva sukham....* (Chandyogya Upanishad 7/23/1)
>
> (Whatever is one with the vast greatness forms the happiness for the person lesser elements of happiness do not imply happiness, the vast, the infinite has to get registered in our consciousness for Bliss—the super joy or intrinsic happiness of life).
>
> *Yatra na anyat pasyati na anyat pasyati na anyat shrunati'N aanyatvijanati'sahbhumah* (Chandyogya Upanishad. 7/24/1)
>
> (Whenever one is focussed on the Supreme oneness of this cosmic creation and not anything else is viewed or heard and known as then he has deviated from the path of realization).

The vast reality of the supreme, the Bhuma, when perceived is actually the underlying and prevailing identity. The process of realization is the process of getting into the realization of the Supreme. *Anahata* opens up the spirit of realization.

Meditation at this level of *anahata chakra* is invoking the open sky and the vastness, clarity of the vast and open sky. After the alternate nostril breathing, concentrating at the level of the centre of the heart and trying to visualize the clear blue sky at the cardiac centre makes the journey upright, leading it higher.

5–7. *Vishudha, Ajna* and *Sahasrara* (the plexuses at throat centre, forehead and top of head): Now, the journey of consciousness up to the level of the cardiac plexus can be discussed. If devotion sets in at the cardiac centre, the force of devotion pushes the consciousness upward for deeper levels of spiritual realization. At the stage of *vishuddha* 16-petalled lotus, that at *ajna chakra* or the forehead plexus four petalled lotus and finally, when the process of realization is complete or it is near completion, thousand petalled lotus gets unfolded. These three are deeply spiritual in nature and the process is absolutely experiential. Spiritual learners should bear a pure mind and a pure heart—a mind that is absolutely detached from all types of gross or subtle desire, fully free from the impacts and influences of ego and largely and solely aimed at divine realization. The person usually develops a spirit of detachment from the impacts of the world. It leads to the disconnect of all relations and all attachments with the world.

The final journey within self-mastery is this process when the mind and intent have become pure, and the person realizes at the core of his being *Chitanandamrupahshivohamaham*.

I am the supreme blissful self; I am embodied with the spirit of ever blissful consciousness—Lord Shiva, within. This journey requires self-initiative towards self-realization. Alternate nostril breathing through *purak, kumbhak* and *rechak* creates a basis to push the consciousness up from the condensed centre at *muladhara* upwards to the top of head for deeper and intense realization.

Required quality of the person for this self-realization is to make the mind simple, *Arjabam* or a simple mind would always create the basis for understanding of the divine consciousness. Simple and steady in the intend to have divine realization facilitate the inner journey. As Patanjali concludes the yoga at the *KaivalyaPada* the oneness:

Purushartha shunyanam gunanam pratiprasavah kaivaly-amswarupprratishthavachitishaktihiti. (Patanjali Yoga 4/34)

(When we have abandoned all other tendencies in life and all attributes are made to coverage to the spirit of divinity, the consciousness of Supreme dawns in the life of people).

Self-realization alone leads to mastery and self-governance.

A realized person attains the quality of true self-leadership. This person is the fittest king, the appropriate personality who makes the right choice in life and activity. The appropriate person, who is capable of leading his own and inner domain, can establish the leadership in such a way that makes the entity undertake the right path of progress. It is thus the spirit within that makes a person realize the Supreme within, brings in and combines the knowledge and expertise of the world to guide and lead any kind of organization in any context. This person becomes a true leader of himself and the organization.

A self-realized person thus creates an internal environment full of divine qualities. He becomes a leader and messenger of noble qualities in the world-gradually creating a society and a system in the world dominated by those noble qualities and thus lead to the creation of a new society and new civilization in the human world. This new civilization will consider every person as equal. The view of life will be one such that divine qualities are present in every person. Therefore, every person is potentially divine. Man will be free from greed, desire, anger, envy, gluttony, selfishness and ego. Man will consider goodness as essential in life and adopt goodness. Truth, integrity, cooperation, selfless work, devotion to the divine, unattached to desires of life, free from meanness, compassionate, caring, friendly to others, helpful to all and supports in the sustenance of life in the world and universe. This man is going to create maintain and foster forward the oncoming divine civilization. The onset of divine civilization shall remove all sorts of poverty, all evils, all vices and clearly establish the VICTORY OF VIRTUE ON EARTH. VIRTUE SHALL WIN.

REFERENCES

Carter, Rita. 2010. *Mapping the Mind*. Chicago: Phoenix Paperbacks

Mukherjee, Siddhartha. 2016. *The Gene: An Intimate History*. London: Penguin Books.

ABOUT THE AUTHOR

Four decades of journey in the pathways of 'management' has made the author engrossed in the spirit of management in both principle and practice. An initial decade as a middle and senior executive and then proceeding to undertake the teaching of 'management' at postgraduate and doctoral levels has created a golden opportunity to realize the limits of the current understanding and focus of 'management'. While delivering lectures at more than a dozen leading universities located in the USA and Europe and many leading institutes and universities in India and the Asian region, the author got the opportunity to learn the mind of learners of the world. On the other hand, a large number of corporate advisories, training and development programmes paved the way to understand the realistic need by the MNCs and large corporations of the days to come. This work is a fruit of those wholesome gains in knowledge and experience.

The author, an MBA, PhD, NET (UGC), with the postdoc work done in Europe, has been awarded numerous international and national awards and accolades, a few of which are as follows:

- 'Dr. Sarvepalli Radhakrishnan Award for Outstanding Contribution to Teaching' from Hindustan Unilever Limited supported by Deloitte and Hexaware
- BBC Knowledge 'Education Leadership Award'
- CIMA (London) global award for 'Outstanding Contributions to Education'
- 'Distinguished Teacher' award by the Department of Business and Economics, Stockholm University, Sweden

- 'Thought Leader Award' at World Education Congress Global Awards for excellence in education, leadership and teaching, presented by CIMA (London)
- 'Visionary Leader Award' received at Fourth Asia's Global Conference held in Singapore

While authoring a large number of publications (books and papers), the focus of the author has been on the spiritual attainment of people. The author has been giving an open discourse on 'Divinity in Life' every Sunday, continuously for the last two decades.

INDEX

Defining stress from holistic
  viewpoint, 7
Degree of autonomy in work, 118
Demand
  hidden or suppressed, 7–8
  perceived, 22
Demands smoothens by
  constraints, 13
Depression and exhaustion, 186
Desire, 52
Devotion, 206
Devotion without distraction,
  206–207
Despair in life, 207
Despondency, 207–208
Different states of mind, 56–59
Dilation of pupils, 201
Direction of transformation, 104
Diseased when predisposed, 76
Dishonest motive, 161–162
  practice, 162
Dis–identification, 43
Distractions, 207
Divine identity of man, 203
Divinity in life, 194–200
Divine Comedy, 178–179
Divine consciousness, 53, 59–60
DNA, 183–184
Doctrine of kosha, 36
Doer as the actor, 77, 80
  as the facilitator, 77
  in a continuum of work, 77
Domain of mind, 56
Dominance factor, 9–13
Doubtful mind, 207
Downsizing strategy, 116
Durant Will, 17
Dyer, 29, 31
Dynamics of stress & coping, 91
Dubos, R., 188

Easwaran, 3–4
Economic deprivation, 70
Ego, 38, 41, 43
Effects of biological conditions,
  186

external situations, 186
stress, 28–32
Ekagra mind, 56–57
Elinor Scarborough, 60
Elliot, T S., 1
Emotions, Social, 208
Emotional energy, xiv
Emotional inclination, 11
Enlargement of the vessels, 201
Envy, 205, 208
Essence of behaviour, 119, 122
Eve, 26
Evolution of consciousness, 172
Exhaustion, 6
Existentialist, 17–18
Expansion of job horizon, 27
Expectations and provisions, 11
Expectancy Valency theory of
  Feather, 73
External pressure, 7, 9
Extrinsic factors to change, 139
Extrinsic Vulnerability, 76

Face the brutes, 16
Factors for human environment,
  118–110
Faith, 205, 207–208
False perception, 207
Fatigue, 189
Feather and Davenport, 73–74
Feather and Bond, 74
  analysis of work structure
    time, 74
Fight, 142, 165, 198
Fire of desire, 52
Five sheaths of existence, 39
Fistula, 191
Flight, 198
Flow of learning in
  organizations, 178
Flow process, 186
  biological conditions, 186
  external situations, 186
Flight, 198
Flow of learning in
  organizations, 178